DROPSY, DIALYSIS, TRANSPLANT

Dropsy, Dialysis, Transplant

A Short History of Failing Kidneys

Steven J. Peitzman

The Johns Hopkins University Press
Baltimore

© 2007 The Johns Hopkins University Press
All rights reserved. Published 2007
Printed in the United States of America on acid-free paper

2 4 6 8 9 7 5 3 1

The Johns Hopkins University Press
2715 North Charles Street
Baltimore, Maryland 21218-4363
www.press.jhu.edu

-

Library of Congress Cataloging-in-Publication Data

Peitzman, Steven J. (Steven Jay), 1945–
Dropsy, dialysis, transplant : a short history of failing kidneys /
Steven J. Peitzman.
p. ; cm. — (Johns Hopkins biographies of disease)
Includes bibliographical references and index.
ISBN-13: 978-0-8018-8734-5 (hardcover : alk. paper)
ISBN-10: 0-8018-8734-8 (hardcover : alk. paper)
1. Chronic renal failure—History. 2. Nephrology—History.
I. Title. II. Series.
[DNLM: 1. Kidney Diseases—history. 2. Nephrology—history.
WJ 11.1 P379d 2007]
RC918.R4P37 2007
616.6′14—dc22   2007013958

A catalog record for this book is available from the British Library.

To the memory of my parents,
Marion and Manuel Peitzman

CONTENTS

Disease is a fundamental aspect of the human condition. Ancient bones tell us that pathological processes are older than humankind's written records, and sickness still confounds our generation's technological pride. We have not banished pain, disability, or the fear of death even if we die, on average at older ages, of chronic and not acute ills, in hospital or hospice beds, and not in our own homes. Disease is something men and women feel. It is something in our bodies—but also in our minds. Disease demands explanation; we think about it and we think with it. Why have I become ill? And why now? How is my body different in sickness from its quiet and unobtrusive functioning in health? Why in times of epidemic has a whole community been scourged?

Answers to such timeless questions necessarily mirror and incorporate available ideas and assumptions. In this sense, disease has always been a social and linguistic as well as biological entity. In the Hippocratic era, physicians—and we have always had them with us—were limited to the evidence of their senses in diagnosing a fever, an abnormal discharge, or seizures. Classical notions of the somatic basis for such alarming symptoms necessarily reflected and expressed contemporary philosophical and physiological notions, a speculative world of disordered humors and "breath." Today we can call for understanding upon a variety of scientific insights and an armory of diagnostic and therapeutic practices—tools that allow us to diagnose ailments unfelt by patients and imperceptible to the doctor's senses. In the past century disease has become increasingly a bureaucratic phenomenon, as well, as sickness has been defined and in that sense constituted by formal disease classifications, treatment protocols, and laboratory thresholds.

Sickness is also linked to climatic and geographic factors. How and where we live and how we distribute our resources all contribute to time- and place-specific incidence of disease. For example, ailments such as typhus fever, plague, malaria, dengue, and yellow fever reflect specific environments that we have shared with our insect contemporaries. But humankind's physical circumstances are determined in part by culture—especially agricultural practice. Environment, demography, ideas, and applied medical knowledge all interact to create particular distributions of disease at particular moments in time. The contemporary ecology of disease in the developed world is marked, for example, by the dominance of chronic and degenerative illness—ailments of the cardiovascular system and of the kidneys, and cancer. And these are ailments neither easily explained and evaded nor managed.

Disease is thus historically as much as biologically specific. Or perhaps I should say that every disease has a unique past. Once discerned and named, every disease claims its own history. At one level biology creates that idiosyncratic identity. Symptoms and epidemiology as well as cultural values and scientific understanding shape responses to illness. Some writers may have romanticized tuberculosis—think of Greta Garbo as Camille—but as the distinguished medical historian Owsei Temkin noted dryly, no one had ever thought to romanticize dysentery. Tuberculosis was pervasive in nineteenth-century Europe and North America and killed far more people than cholera did, but it never mobilized the same widespread and policy-shifting anxiety. Unlike tuberculosis, cholera killed quickly and dramatically and was never accepted as a condition of life. Sporadic cases of influenza are normally invisible, indistinguishable among a variety of respiratory infections; waves of epidemic flu are all too visible. Syphilis and other sexually transmitted diseases, to cite another example, have had a peculiar and morally inflected attitudinal history. Some diseases, such as smallpox or malaria, have a long history; others, like AIDS, have a rather short one. Some have flourished under modern conditions; others seem to reflect the realities of an earlier and less economically developed world.

These arguments constitute the logic motivating the Johns Hopkins Biographies of Disease. Biography implies a coherent identity, a chronology, and a narrative—a movement in and through time. Once inscribed by name in our collective understanding of medicine, each disease entity becomes a part of that collective understanding and, thus, inevitably shapes the way in which individuals think about their own felt symptoms and prospects for future health. Each historically visible entity—each disease—has a distinct history, even if that history is not always defined in terms familiar to twenty-first century physicians. Dropsy and Bright's Disease are no longer terms of everyday clinical practice, but they are an integral part of the history of chronic kidney disease.

Steven Peitzman's biography of such ills begins with pain and disability—with phenomena felt by patients and described by physicians. It begins with watery swellings—dropsy—and with weakness and premature death. Today's kidney disease is a very different entity. It is an ailment mediated by a century and a half of increasing physiological understanding and a growing capacity for highly technical interventions—most conspicuously dialysis and transplantation. It is also a history of bureaucracy, of the shaping of individual lives by blood chemistry readings. An elevated creatinine level legitimates a diagnosis of chronic or acute kidney failure and thus dialysis, perhaps hospital admission, and—in the United States—Medicare reimbursement.

If disease exists both inside the individual patient's body and mind and outside of the particular sufferer's body in the form of collectively agreed-upon understandings and practices, then no ailment represents that sociological truth more sharply than the protagonist of this biography. Bright's Disease was probably the first doctor's disease, in the sense of being named after its discoverer. In the 1820s, Richard Bright, an English physician and pathologist, linked clinical symptoms and chemical findings (albumen in the patient's urine) during life with characteristic appearances of kidney pathology after death—thus "creating" that eponymous disease entity called Bright's Disease. That construction and, in a sense, expropriation of the suffering patient's experience are characteristic of a more general trend in Western medicine, the growing dominance of specific disease concepts organized around an underlying mechanism—whether a characteristic lesion or pathologically altered physiological process. One might in fact argue that we have entered a new phase in which the boundaries between individual and collective, internal and external, and body and available technology seem to be breaking down.

Medical ideas have always had an impact on individual patients: think of the centuries during which men and women were bled and purged in accordance with accepted notions of disease causation. But with dialysis and transplant, the body has become increasingly permeable, increasingly susceptible to re-engineering. The history of kidney disease is in this sense both the biography of a persistent human nemesis and at the same time a metaphor for more general trends. The reader can decide whether the burden of this narrative is progressive and utopian or grimly dystopian. But in either case, the story illustrates the capacity of disease at once to constitute and illuminate the human condition.

Charles E. Rosenberg

PREFACE

No one, it seems, writes songs about the kidney. Compared to the heart, brain, or even liver, the kidney attracts only scant interest or respect. Many persons are not quite sure where in the body the kidneys reside, and I suspect that a few do not know that each of us ordinarily owns a pair of them. Almost everyone has a general sense of what they do—produce a certain unappreciated fluid that is usually disposed of as quickly and quietly as possible. Whereas most people can identify the work of the cardiologist or dermatologist, "nephrologist"—a specialist in diseases of the kidney—is a term little recognized, and difficult to spell or pronounce. The common adjective that refers to the kidney, "renal," is also relatively unknown—perhaps it turns up in crossword puzzles. Yet one cannot live without kidneys, which filter from the blood and discharge in the urine a variety of potentially toxic bodily wastes. The kidneys also regulate very precisely the body's contents of sodium, water, and potassium; adjust the acidity of the blood; stimulate the production of red blood cells; take part in setting the blood pressure; and contribute to the well-being of bones. Thus, disease of the kidney can result in a wide range of symptoms, and loss of their normal functioning can lead to death.

This book will not deal with all diseases to which the kidney is subject: readers won't encounter discussions of urinary tract infections, rare inherited disorders, cancers, or even the very common and notoriously painful kidney stone. Rather, I have chosen to focus on what might be called the set of generalized, often progressive, disorders that cause the common finding called "proteinuria" (the leakage of blood proteins into the urine by faulty renal filtering) and that can lead in many patients to overall failure of the kidney's excretory ability. When this occurs, the buildup of certain normally present bodily substances to toxic levels produces the complex of symptoms called "uremia." It includes loss of appetite

xiii

and vomiting, itching of the skin, chest pains, fatigue, and—if untreated—seizure, coma, and death. In addition, the failure of kidney function can lead to the accumulation of salt and water in the body, which physicians once called "dropsy" and now refer to as "edema." Indeed, it was through the care and careful study of dropsical patients that British physician Richard Bright in the 1820s through 1840s was able to associate fluid retention with proteinuria, the uremic symptoms, and the finding of diseased kidneys at autopsy. "Bright's Disease" soon became the widely accepted term for proteinuric renal disease as a category. It remained a recognized and useful term until about 1950, and I use it in this book, sometimes perhaps playfully, even when discussing later periods.

This book joins others in a series called Johns Hopkins Biographies of Disease, and I have tried to take that concept seriously. In one sense, diseases exist only in people or animals: there are no independently existing cases of pneumonia floating about in the air. In another sense, however, diseases do exist in the abstract, as concepts to be established, understood, written about, and of course diagnosed and treated in individuals. Following the work of series editor Charles E. Rosenberg, I discuss Bright's Disease (under various names) as a "being" with a kind of "agency"— meaning, a power to do things in the world, as human subjects of actual biographies might. Similarly, I try to place the "life" of this disease within the changing customs, ideas, and practices of medicine and the broader world. In general, I describe a trend by which the illness interacts with an increasingly complex cast of characters including of course patients, doctors, and nurses, but also governments, corporations, foundations, and the media.

But why (one might reasonably ask) write a book on the history of kidney disease at all? First, there is a lot of it: by the year 2000, something like one million persons worldwide whose kidneys were destroyed by disease stayed alive through treatments with hemodialysis (the artificial kidney) or kidney transplantation—and this number represents only those patients with the most severe or "end-stage" phase of the disorder. Proteinuric renal disease can be caused by other maladies ranging from diabetes to malaria to AIDS, and no region of the world seems free of it. It is known that renal failure is particularly common in Japan, Spain, Taiwan, and the United States. Second, a narrative of the history of kidney disease provides an excellent way to trace changes in how diseases have been defined, categorized, understood, and treated. Thus for Bright's Disease one can see stages in which it was defined by its symptoms, then by pathology (structural changes in the organ) together with the laboratory (analysis of blood and urine). Eventually, understanding was sought in research centers, down to the molecular and genetic level by the late twentieth century. In the 1990s, however, some physicians interested in kidney disease embraced a new epidemiological approach that stressed populations and prevention. Third, the story of kidney disease and kidney failure includes two remarkable innovations, which symbolize modern technological medicine and surgery—the artificial kidney and transplantation. In fact, the artificial kidney (hemodialysis) can claim standing as the first routinely successful organ replacement device, while the first widely performed internal organ transplantation was that of the kidney. Seemingly at the other extreme, however, the ancient modality of diet therapy has at times played a major role in the treatment of kidney disease, and still holds a place. Also since antiquity, doctors have prescribed and patients ingested medicines, and these as well enter into the stories of dropsy and of kidneys in trouble. In fact, the expenditures for drugs by or for patients with chronic kidney disease in the early twenty-first century easily amounts to several billion dollars in the United States alone—I could find no accurate figure.

The history of kidney disease also provides an excellent tool for exploring the experience of illness in successive time periods, including being diagnosed and being treated. Why might such exploration be of value? If nothing else, sickness has always formed a part of human life, and usually the pathway to its end. It is therefore a just subject for historical analysis and presentation. In addition, the future of medical care will undoubtedly see an increasing variety of technologic treatments and transplantations. Thus, understanding the personal experience of persons who are joined three times weekly to a dialysis machine, and those who have received a kidney transplant or sometimes two, may prove

useful in anticipating the responses and emotional needs of patients who will receive new but similar therapeutic interventions. I
hope, of course, that some patients and members of their families
will read this book in order to learn something about the history
of the disease that has altered their lives. In an attempt to make
the volume more useful to patients, I have for the early chapters
added a section called "A Later Perspective" that relates the historical background to current thought and practice. Of course, this
information will itself in due course become historical, as ideas
and therapeutics further evolve.

This volume is not mainly a history of nephrology as a specialty within medicine, so readers will find little detail about its
organizations, certifying boards, and the like. I have, however,
written and published on the history of American nephrology as
a specialty elsewhere, and use some of that work here.[1] Certainly
physicians and surgeons who have nurtured a special interest and
expertise in renal disease and its treatments will appear throughout the chapters. But they will not outnumber the patients, who
include a novelist, laborers in nineteenth-century London, a double Nobel Prize recipient, and a star of professional basketball.
In chapters 7 and 8, I develop the idea that the modern recipient of chronic hemodialysis treatment or a kidney transplantation
has become a career patient, herself or himself a sort of specialist
within the universe of patients. ("Chronic hemodialysis" refers to
repeated treatments with an artificial kidney, usually three times
each week, to replace irreversibly destroyed kidney function, and
thereby keep alive a person with this devastating loss.)

I have devoted but scant space to investigation of kidney function and disease in the research laboratory, especially for the period from the mid-twentieth century until the present (2007 as I
write this). Adequately developing an account of such research,
including the recent trends in molecular understanding, would
prove an enormous task best tackled by someone who has been
engaged in such work.[2]

Although this book is not a history of nephrologists, I have allowed the clinician part of me a place in it, clearly not as a major
figure in the field (which I am not), but rather more as an internal
observer of its past and present. That is, I have tried in several

places to offer what insights and interpretations I can as an historian who is also a practitioner in the area of renal disease. In doing so, I use the first-person voice more than is commonly done in historical works of this sort.

The chapters dealing with the later twentieth century and twenty-first century center largely on events and persons in the United States, particularly as I explore the growth of chronic dialysis and kidney transplantation and the experiences of those benefiting from these treatments. This emphasis reflects my area of greatest knowledge and interest (or said another way, my limitations as an historian and linguist), and recognizes that most readers of this book will be North Americans. Beyond this, it is the case that chronic dialysis began in the United States (though the artificial kidney was not invented here), and some of the most important early efforts at renal transplantation took place there and in Canada. Nonetheless, I do not doubt that what I offer is a very incomplete account. Many subjects warrant more than one sort of biography, and such likely will be the case for kidney disease as its prevalence becomes better known. I hope this volume proves a useful introduction to the most serious disorders of an organ of indispensable biological importance, even if it is not the stuff of poetry.

ACKNOWLEDGMENTS

I have been studying and writing about the history of kidney disease and the specialty nephrology for about thirty years. This book marks a culmination of that work, though it by no means merely compiles past efforts. Still, these acknowledgments will reflect on my earlier studies as well as the present volume.

Of course, I have used many libraries and archival collections, most indispensably the magnificent Library of the College of Physicians of Philadelphia. I have also consulted books and documents at the Library of the American Philosophical Society, Guy's Hospital, the National Library of Medicine, Oregon State University Libraries, Stanford University Library, the Van Pelt Library of the University of Pennsylvania, the Library of the Medical College of Pennsylvania, and the Wellcome Institute for the History of Medicine. I am much in debt to staff members of these institutions. Research grants that secured time for historical research and sometimes paid for travel came helpfully from the National Endowment for the Humanities, the National Library of Medicine, and the American Philosophical Society.

Some of the ideas in this volume, and even a few of the sentences, appeared first in my essay "From Bright's Disease to End-Stage Renal Disease," which appeared in the anthology *Framing Disease: Studies in Cultural History,* edited by Charles E. Rosenberg and Janet Golden (New Brunswick, N.J.: Rutgers University Press, 1992). That collection grew out of a conference supported by the Milbank Memorial Fund and the Wood Institute for the History of Medicine of the College of Physicians of Philadelphia. Of course, I also draw upon other of my published articles, which are cited in the end notes.

Anyone who seeks to write about the history of disease walks in particular pathways created by other historians, and I hope I have honored, by attaining something more than imitation, Charles E. Rosenberg (my teacher since my college years at Penn) and Roy Porter, whom I knew mainly through his books. My friend Russell C. Maulitz has over many years helped shape my thinking about the pasts of pathology and internal medicine. Many historians and graduate students of the Department of the History and Sociology of Science at the University of Pennsylvania have welcomed me to their shop for over twenty years and helped me try to think like an historian. Corinna Schlombs, when a graduate student at that department, carried out some research for me the results of which reshaped the later part of the book. Other colleagues in history who have contributed to the genesis of this book include Toby Appel and Thomas Horrocks. Nephrologists and other clinicians who have kindly answered questions about their work or helped me in other ways include Barry Brenner, J. Stewart Cameron, Garabed Eknoyan, George Schreiner, Belding Scribner, and the late Carl Gottschalk. Christine Ruggere helped me with my exploration of Richard Bright's *Reports of Medical Cases* as a book and colored atlas. The anonymous readers for the Johns Hopkins University Press provided several good suggestions.

Colleagues and trainees in the nephrology division of The Medical College of Pennsylvania (now that of Drexel University College of Medicine) have over the years tolerated my numerous historical interjections at our conferences and on rounds, and have expressed interest when I presented some of my work to them more formally. Many of my patients over the years have made clear the importance of including the experience of the sick, including their courage and tolerance, in a work such as this. One patient kindly allowed me to photograph him during one of his hemodialysis treatments. More recently, my new employer (for part of my time), the Educational Commission for Foreign Medical Graduates, its senior officers and human resources staff, proved typically collegial in permitting me a brief leave of absence.

A most essential person in my life, Nancy Pontone, was a careful reader of drafts and cheered me on with excessive praise. Her skilled niece, science illustrator Elisheva Marcus, provided an elegant rendering of the nephron.

As with any author dealing with her, I am indebted to the collaboration and good sense of Jacqueline Wehmueller, Executive Editor at the Johns Hopkins University Press. I offer thanks as well to other staff at the Press, and to copy editor Michael Baker.

DROPSY, DIALYSIS, TRANSPLANT

CHAPTER ONE

Swollen with Dropsy

—⟨≈⟩—

This small book will tell the history of kidney disease, or at least some of its forms. But the prehistory of kidney disease was dropsy. John Wesley, founder of Methodism and medical author, told the countless readers of his *Primitive Physic* that dropsy was "a preter-natural collection of water in the head, breast, belly, or all over the body. It is attended with a continual thirst. The part swelled pits if you press it with your fingers. The urine is pale and little." A physician of the fourteenth century, John of Gaddesden, had de-scribed it simply as "a watery disease inflating the body," though he wrote in Latin and called the disorder "idropisis."[1]

Persons have suffered this suffocating and frightening watery swelling since the earliest days of recorded medicine—and no doubt before—and have done so all over the world. Since the time of Hippocrates, medical students have learned to pinch with fingers at the ankle, diligently testing for dropsy of the legs. Both medical attendant and patient might note that as the water builds up in legs and belly, so its flow as outgoing urine decreases (as Wesley knew), though not all dropsy originates from kidney disease. Some adverse factor that limits the kidneys' capacity to dump water, however, always plays a role (in current understand-ing): dropsy occurs when the kidneys are diseased, or—as will be seen later—deceived by a diseased liver or heart.

Anyway, it's fair to begin a book about the history of kidney diseases with dropsy. (Dropsy of the abdominal cavity was and is called "ascites," and that of the limbs, "edema." The sum of these in extreme degree owns the melodious name "anasarca.")

—◦◦◦—

An illustration from a German medical text of 1695 shows one comprehensively dropsical person (she qualifies for anasarca).[2] A forty-eight-year-old mother of five children, she was an actual patient, induced, or simply caused, to have her misery depicted and documented by the woodcutter's art. What do we see in this striking portrait of sickness? The patient is a woman, and that is not by chance: over the hundreds of years that dropsy was seen as a disease, medical authorities (such as the seventeenth-century British physician Thomas Sydenham) wrote that "women are more subject to it than men." (This may have merely been because huge, fluid-filled ovarian cysts that once afflicted women were confused with, or accepted as one category of, dropsy.)[3] She sits up in a chair, though sick persons usually are portrayed reclining in bed. Yielding one's accustomed activities and taking to bed have long marked the transition from health to serious illness. The dropsical person, however, cannot easily lie down, for the mass of fluid distending the abdomen would press up on the lungs, cutting off breath—even if the lungs themselves were not yet suffused with water, or surrounded by fluid collections in the thorax. So "asthma" (meaning at one time merely "shortness of breath") often joined dropsy; and the victim—such as an eighteenth-century patient of British doctor William Withering—sits "supported upright in his chair, by pillows, every attempt to lean back or stoop forward giving him the sensation of instantaneous suffocation."[4]

Neither could the patient much get out of the chair to move around. Enormous extra work is involved in carrying the weight of the dropsy, often easily fifty pounds or more. The muscles can barely move the legs, and the effort triggers the breathlessness. The unused muscles wither, even if the underlying disease has not directly injured them. So the dropsical person was often confined to home, or in periods later than our woodcut, to hospital, and at most extreme, confined to life in a chair (this will be replayed centuries later, in the days of dialysis). And yet, for the affluent sufferer, we shall see that dropsy sometimes had the power to dic-

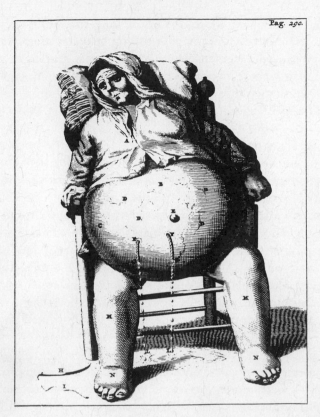

A woman with dropsy, showing the procedure of "tapping," or paracentesis, from Frederik Dekkers, *Exercitationes Practicae circa Medendi Methodum* (Leyden, 1695). Courtesy of the Library of the College of Physicians of Philadelphia.

tate that the patient travel—to a warmer climate, for dropsy was a disease long linked to cold, and treated by sweating, among other remedies.

The ill woman in the drawing wears only a blouse and some sort of bonnet—perhaps she remains otherwise unclothed for better visibility of the enormously engorged abdomen and the fluid-filled legs. Maybe none of her clothing can now be fit upon her. The bonnet offers a futile token of female modesty. Her face does not meet the gaze of the onlooker but rather seems disengaged, grim, resigned, or sunk in lassitude. She has, however, agreed, probably in desperation, to one of the longest continuously used mechanical treatments in medicine—her belly has been "tapped." A curving needle (shown near her right foot) guiding a sort of string, or wick, was inserted through the abdominal wall and out again, creating passageways by which the trapped dropsical fluid might escape. We see it dripping onto the floor and even splashing a bit.

Surgeons in the ancient Greek world reportedly tapped the abdomen to drain dropsy (or ascites).[5] John of Gaddesden described the procedure in his *Rosa Anglica,* a medical treatise written in the late 1300s and first printed in the fifteenth century. John recommended a technique different from that in our illustration: a puncture might be made "three fingers' breadth below the umbilicus" but oblique in its passage through the several abdominal layers, then the water is allowed to escape—not all at once!—through an inserted "cannula made of gold or silver or bronze."[6]

Serious disease, of course, holds personal and social meaning. Some of this we have already inferred for the illustrated dropsical woman—she has necessarily withdrawn from whatever her normal activities may have been, into the chair. Seeing her as she appears in the drawing, others would respond with empathy, pity, horror—-possibly even disgust. She is bloated and beached, grotesque. The abdomen, which in a woman might be fruitfully engorged with child, now contains only water, which must be caused to drip onto the floor; she is entirely unable even to place a basin below to catch it. Another of the common chronic diseases known through the ages—consumption (accepted to mean, usually, tuberculosis), shrank a woman, increased her delicacy, created a perhaps refined pallor. And—this is a long-held cultural belief—consumption might even arouse creativity and romantic passion. But not dropsy: no one thought it improved one's looks, or amorous potential. Andrew Jackson, rugged battlefield warrior and seventh president of the United States, who died massively dropsical, said of himself in his last days: "I am a blubber of water."[7]

Furthermore, since ancient times dropsy has been deemed a companion to inebriety. The Athenian writer Philostratus wrote of a youth who lived a life of luxury: "[D]rink was his life, or rather his death, for in fact he had dropsy and from love of wine neglected a dry diet." Thomas Sydenham, the "English Hippocrates," in 1683 taught that "great drinkers are most subject to the dropsy"; and William Cullen, possibly the leading English-speaking physician of the late eighteenth century, listed "intemperance in use of intoxicating liquors as one cause among many." William Buchan, the eighteenth-century progenitor of the immensely popular *Domestic Medicine* believed that dropsy "may likewise proceed from drinking ardent spirits, or other strong liquors. It is true, almost to a proverb, that great drinkers die of dropsy." In an 1823 memoir of captivity among North American Indians, one writer seemed to observe that dropsy occurred among the Native Americans "who had become intemperate by their intercourse with the whites."[8] The connection of intemperance with dropsy was endlessly repeated in medical writings both for professional and lay readers, though how pervasive was the idea in the popular mind one cannot know. But at least in some times and places, the sufferer from dropsy risked being thought an inebriate. Swollen, useless, sometimes messily weeping water across the tense skin of the turgid legs, or spouting it through a burst abdomen—and perhaps suspect of having brought it all on oneself through drunkenness— the dropsical person was a miserable vessel of watery sickness and torment.

"MY DISEASES ARE AN ASTHMA AND A DROPSY": SAMUEL JOHNSON

To gain some firsthand sense of the experience of dropsy, we can read the letters of an extraordinary reporter. In the last year of his celebrated life, writer and lexicographer Samuel Johnson (1709–1784) suffered with asthma (meaning shortness of breath, not the disease now labeled with this term) and dropsy, and told of the experience to his doctors, to his biographer James Boswell, and to other friends. Already troubled by periods of breathlessness, his legs began to swell during the fall and early winter of 1783–1784. Like many knowledgeable persons with dropsy, he perceived that "the season is a great part of my disease, and that when warm weather restores perspiration, the watery disease will evaporate," or so he was "at least willing to flatter" himself.[9] Indeed, old persons with chronic illness living in colder climates have long wondered if each winter might be their last. But ancient tradition held dropsy to be a disease specifically connected to the cold humor "phlegm" and to chill-induced suppression of that salutary perspiration so essential to the body's economy. On February 11, 1784—now deep into winter and confined to his London home—Johnson wrote to Boswell: "The asthma, however, is not the worst. A dropsy gains ground upon me; my legs and thighs are very much swollen with water, which I should be content if I could keep it there, but I am afraid it will soon be higher."[10] And it soon was.

Then in late February of 1784 a remarkable event relieved Dr. Johnson's pulmonary and peripheral edemas: "Last week I emitted in about twenty hours, full twenty pints of urine, and the tumour of my body is very much lessened, but whether the water will not gather again, He only knows by whom we live and move."[11] Johnson wrote to everyone about this mighty post-devotional discharge of fluid, and Boswell included it in the *Life of Samuel Johnson,* making it unquestionably the most famous diuresis in the history of the English-speaking peoples. The great writer and dictionary maker, a man much attuned to science and rationalism, assigned the intervention to the Divine. Still too ill to leave home, he was grateful for being again able to dress himself, to button stockings and trousers around once-more recognizable knees and belly. Johnson's suffering was, however, not over. Toward spring, he did venture out—not south, but north, to his familiar country retreat in his native Derbyshire, to "try what air and regularity will effect."[12] But, on July 21 he wrote to one of his physicians: "The water has in these summer months made two invasions, but has run off again with no very formidable tumefaction."[13]

Into late summer (which refused to get warm) and early fall, armed with squills and cantharides (medications then considered diuretics), Johnson battled the floods, which would rise and fall. Shortness of breath continued to torment him, as well as sleeplessness at night and weakness of his legs, though he sustained some improvement through a good part of August. By early September, his "[w]ater has again run away," his breath "no longer distressfully strait," and he could finally sleep in bed, rather than sitting up, in the posture of dropsy.[14] In October he admitted to a friend that "[m]y diseases are an Asthma and a Dropsy, and, what is less curable, seventy five."[15] Not surprisingly, this distinguished poet of a maritime island nation described the ups and downs of his ravaged, volatile body with the language of floods and seas. Two days later he wrote (to Dr. Brocklesby), "The water encreases almost visibly and the squills which I get here [Lichfield] are utterly inefficacious. My spirits are extremely low. Yet I have recovered from a worse state."[16]

His spirits were low: he felt awful, had lost control over the contours and workings of his body, and now could not get out of his Derbyshire home. Missing the sustenance of lively conversation, he felt intensely the isolation of the very ill—"In this place," he had written on August 14 to a friend, "I have everything but company, and of company I am in great want."[17] The letters of his friends enlivened his miserable and sedentary days and nights, whereas his outgoing correspondence dwelt much on his illnesses. Dealing with them by now formed his primary occupation. Serving as his own on-site physician, he desperately pressed use of the squills as a diuretic, and of opiates to ease his breathing. "Relapsing into the dropsy very fast," in early November of 1784 he prepared to return to London.[18]

—⟞⟐⟐⟞—

Johnson succumbed on December 13, 1784, and the autopsy revealed both cardiac and renal disease (the heart dilated and thickened, the right kidney atrophic, the left cystic). But in life Johnson, like many similarly afflicted, had dropsy, not kidney failure or congestive heart failure, concepts of a later age. The experience of his disease was dreadful: a constant struggle against the drowning of his body by floodwaters from within, a struggle waged with drugs he knew to be inadequate, unpredictable, and noxious. The immobility brought on by the dropsy and asthma robbed him of the club life and other social settings his mind and spirit so demanded, though from his dropsy chair he could maintain his vigorous correspondence, and through it, the regard and affection of his friends. If any of them thought that his dropsy was brought on by a lifetime of excessive indulgence in good food and drink, surely none saw any value in saying so. On one momentous occasion, following prayer and fasting, a capricious deity seemed to provide him with a miraculous reprieve, in the form of a great flow of urine. Maybe this event, even if it made no lasting cure, boosted his faith in God, which would have given some comfort, since it is known that he much feared death. Dropsy sometimes was cured, or at least for long periods the waters could be stayed. But it was a dangerous ailment: as wrote William Heberden, one of Johnson's physicians, "[W]hen persons after having laboured for some time under the complaints of the lungs, or of the bowels, begin to find a swelling in the legs, it is a sign of some deep mischief in the breast or abdomen, the swelling will most probably increase to a just dropsy, and the case end fatally."[19]

MEDICAL IDEAS ON THE CAUSES AND TREATMENT OF DROPSY

In contemporary medicine, a clear distinction is made between *diseases,* and their manifestations, or *symptoms.* Thus, asthma, malaria, heart attack, and hepatitis count as diseases, with shortness of breath, fever, chest pain, jaundice some of their symptoms. Sometimes, physicians conceive of an intermediary process of disturbed bodily function (the pathophysiology): the "disease" myocardial infarction (heart attack) has led to the process "congestive heart failure" (which can be caused also by other heart diseases), and the findings that the patient or doctor can perceive include shortness of breath, fatigue, crackling sounds in the lungs, and a "gallop" rhythm to the heart sounds. During the two thousand years or so during which "dropsy" existed as a sickness and a diagnosis in Western medicine, these distinctions (among "disease," "pathophysiology," and "symptom") held less meaning. Dropsy was largely looked upon as a disease, in our sense, though it was certainly proposed by some physicians that it was something like a consequence of a more primary derangement elsewhere, such as in the liver (more on this later).

As a disease it was a common and serious one and was discussed in writings from the Hippocratic treatises through the nineteenth century. All experienced physicians would encounter it, and surgeons were called in when a patient needed "paracentesis," or the tapping of fluid out of the abdominal cavity. Even before seeing a practitioner, persons could easily recognize dropsical swelling and seek some aid through popular remedy books and health guides or the almanacs that became widely and cheaply available, particularly in the United States. Though treatable and occasionally curable, dropsy consistently turns up as a cause of death, even if it always ranked behind fevers, consumption, and diarrhea or the other mishaps of childhood. This is seen from the seventeenth century through the beginning of the nineteenth century in the mortality bills of London, and similarly in other cities of Europe.[20] In Philadelphia, even during the horrific Yellow Fever year of 1793, among the families of the parish of Christ Church (and the allied St. Peter's Church), where 214 were carried off by the epidemic, still 9 parishioners died from dropsy. Medical historian J. Worth Estes concluded that a fairly stable 2 to 5 percent of deaths in Britain and the United States since the seventeenth century has been attributed to dropsy (which Estes chooses to virtually equate retroactively with congestive heart failure, a supposition that might be challenged).[21]

Medical writers consistently over hundreds of years listed as the symptoms and signs of dropsy the obvious swelling with fluid, the pitting left after pressing on the ankle, thirst, rapid heart rate, shortness of breath, and decreased urinary output. Physicians reached consensus for these observations. But only with much less agreement could they attempt to understand the causes and meaning of dropsy within the prevalent medical theories of their time.[22] Beginning with the writings traditionally associated with the Greek physician Hippocrates, and assigned to the fourth and fifth centuries BC, the four "humors" and four "qualities" would dominate medical thought through something like the seventeenth century, both in European and Arabic medicine. Health and deviation from it depended upon the proper balance and purity of the four humors—blood, phlegm, yellow bile, and black bile. Each of these owned specific properties (yellow bile was "hot and dry," phlegm "cold and wet"), and each was associated with a major organ (the liver for yellow bile, the brain for phlegm). There is neither space nor need to explore the details of this system here; suffice it to say that as spun out and expanded, especially by the Graeco-Roman physician and anatomist Galen (AD 130–201), the humoral system became a versatile and comprehensive framework, able to answer most questions early physicians raised about disease and therapy. At the same time, it avoided rigidity, and within it there existed ample room for enjoyable debate and conjecture. Furthermore, it could be joined to a more anatomical focus on particular organs as the seat of diseases, as favored at various times by particular sects or "schools" of physicians.

Most of the references to dropsy in the Hippocratic writings offer brief points of advice concerning diagnosis and prognosis. The more theoretical Galen, within his vast writings, generally saw dropsy as a disease of the liver (other ancient authorities favored the spleen) but also allowed that excess of the phlegm, the most watery and "cold" of humors, could produce a dropsy. As the system of humors and qualities devolved into a simpler and more practical form during the Middle Ages, dropsy became mostly linked to phlegm, particularly when in excess, spilling downward from the brain to the belly, but most importantly with the quality of cold. That dropsy could follow exposure to a chill—especially when one was drunk—assumed the status of fact, or even natural law, and physicians seemed to see the rule played out regularly in their practices. This rule endured long after the demise of the formal humoral system.[23]

By the seventeenth century, newer anatomical and even mechanistic, or physiological, concepts prevailed in European medicine. Now, dropsy could be seen as a disorder of the proper generation of blood, or of its "strength." If the watery component of imperfectly made blood could too readily separate from its other parts and leak out of the vascular system into the legs and abdomen, dropsy would result. Or, the mechanism might be seen as some dynamic imbalance between the "exhalant" systems of the body and its "absorbent" functions, the balance of which determined the amount of fluid that should reside in various bodily locations. These disordered processes in turn might be caused by such mishaps as liver disease, fevers, dysenteries, excess bloodletting, suppression of menstruation, bad diet, and—as already noted—intemperance and exposure to cold. A particular author might list a dozen other remote causes of dropsical swelling, so many in fact, that the meaning of "causes" vanishes for the modern reader.

But identifying the originating cause no doubt sometimes did matter: in order to prevent recurrence, the physician could advise a change in diet, the avoidance of cold beverages, less alcohol, and so on. It is more difficult to estimate the practical value of the changing notions of what we might call the mechanism of dropsy or the theory of its formation (and these I have described above only very sketchily). Probably the theory a practitioner favored would, at times, help guide therapy, but more likely the formulation and deliberation of such ideas meant more to the physician than the patient. This would be the case especially for physicians (of any period) who saw medicine as part of the natural sciences, diseases as a part of the natural world that could be studied and understood. Also, the possession of theoretical knowledge marked the well-bred physician of the upper strata, an always desirable distinction. Beyond this, thinking about, even debating, competing ideas gives intellectual pleasure, which might balance the often mundane repetition of daily medical life, or of any professional work.

Men and women who are ill desire relief, not mechanistic concepts, and their physicians have always needed to deliver. Patients with dropsy, simply put, need to get rid of the water. Fortunately, the medications Western physicians had been using for virtually *all* ailments from antiquity until the nineteenth century, did exactly that. With a basis in old humoral ideas, or in notions of disease-causing substances in need of removal from the body, they relied on purgatives, emetics, sudorifics (drugs to induce sweating, also called diaphoretics), and diuretics, or at least drugs believed to be diuretics. When using these drugs for dropsy, the physician's objective was more directly to carry excess fluid out of the body, one way or another. No appeal was needed to a mishap of the humors, or the need to eject some "moribific" influence. Domestic medicine books such as William Buchan's and passages in popular almanacs listed the same remedies for dropsy that learned physicians recommended in their texts for the profession.[24] Thus, through prescription or on their own, dropsical persons before 1900 took vegetable laxatives such as "jalap" and "elaterium," and extracts of the dwarf elder shrub (or tree), and many other time-honored remedies that purged, puked, or sweated.

Emetics or "vomitives" had their particular place in treating dropsy. The notable British physician Thomas Sydenham (1624–

1689) in 1682 saw a "poor woman" of fifty-five years who had been suffering from an "intermittent fever, and afterwards lain in prison three years: she had suffered much from cold, and her belly was more swelled than I had ever seen any person's before." He treated her with a vomitive, "crocus metallorum," a salt of the metal antimony. It worked, and "after the third dose the swelling began to fall, and in a fortnight her belly appeared to be shrunk a yard, by the thread with which I had ordered it to be measured at first, and she assured me that she had voided several gallons of water." The antimony seemed to have worked first as an emetic, then as a diuretic. She could now lay her head on a pillow "and turn from side to side as she pleased." But the repeated vomits "raised the vapours so much, as to render their further use unsafe." She still showed some fullness of the abdomen and "pits in the legs" when anything was pressed against them, so Sydenham followed with his "purging potion," which contained, among other ingredients, "berries of the buckthorn." For other patients, Sydenham used preparations of the broom plant, a supposed diuretic, to discharge the burden of water through the urine.[25]

As we already acknowledged, the numerous purgatives and laxatives were not at all specific remedies for dropsy, being given—and taken—for a wide range of ailments; diuretics and sudorifics perhaps enjoyed more limited and focused use. This seemingly noxious, and of course sickening, reliance on such measures over the centuries speaks to how embedded these practices were in Western medicine and how largely they were accepted and in meaningful ways understood by both patient and doctor. Both could see an immediate demonstration of something happening, a sign that an act of doctoring, a therapeutic alteration, had indeed occurred.[26]

Dropsical patients were willing to trade the awful nausea and retching, and the cumbersome appeals to the bedpan or chamber pot, for some hope of getting out of the chair, of seeing the contour of the body return to a recognizable outline. And some did enjoy improvement, because at least for many, the treatments clearly worked. From our twenty-first-century perspective, we consider that the loss of water and salts through drug-induced vomiting and diarrhea would first diminish the fluid portion of blood (the source of the secreted stomach and intestinal fluids) in such a way that gradually, and with repetition of the doses, the salt and water forming the dropsy would find their way back into the bloodstream to make up the losses. Then this "mobilized" fluid itself will go out through the stomach or bowels with further dosing.[27] It is therefore possible that dropsy played a lasting role in proving the value and sustaining the use of the emetics and purgatives that formed the underpinning of pharmaceutical treatment of disease for over fifteen hundred years. For whatever we might think about their use in fever, hysteria, convulsions, or headache, for dropsy, the plan often succeeded. It reduced total body salt and water, and—at least for a time—the waters did recede.

Dropsy, however, holds the distinction of being the object of treatment by a medication that represented something new in medical care and notable in its literature. It was announced in the late eighteenth century and is still with us today. In 1785 British physician William Withering (1741–1799) published his *Account of the Foxglove,* a careful analysis of almost ten years' experience treating dropsy with extract of the foxglove plant, or *Digitalis purpurea.* He had heard of it first as a "secret" remedy used by "an old woman in Shropshire who had sometimes made cures after the more regular practitioners had failed," but he came to learn that it was known in other rural areas.[28] Yorkshire people "often cure themselves of dropsical complaints by drinking Foxglove tea."[29]

Withering's book comprises a series of case descriptions—an old and honored genre of medical writing—followed by some conclusions and advice. Case number 20 is typical. The man presented with "Hydrops Pectoris" (fluid in the chest), with "legs and thighs prodigiously anasarcous" and "a very distressing sense of fulness [*sic*] and tightness across his stomach." His breath was short and urine output scant. His situation worsened despite "various medicine" and "blistering." Withering prescribed an infusion (i.e., a solution in water) of digitalis. It "made him very sick" (presumably, he became nauseated and vomited) but "acted powerfully as a diuretic, and removed all his symptoms." But about three months later, Mr. H_____ was "out upon a journey, and after taking cold, was suddenly seized with difficulty breathing." Before the full dropsy could recur, digitalis was again utilized, with relief.[30] Case 73, seen in June of 1781, like many who Withering treated, was "a hard drinker," afflicted with "asthma, jaundice, and dropsy." His appetite was "gone," his urine "foul and in small quantity." Various conventional medicines had failed, but an infusion of digitalis leaves "acted powerfully as a diuretic, and removed the most urgent of his complaints, viz, the dropsical and asthmatical symptoms."[31] This man's breathing grew worse the following winter; he died, but without recurrence of dropsy.

Withering's cases (162 in all) reveal the foxglove to have been remarkably successful, for about two-thirds of the patients, in working as a diuretic to relieve the dropsy and frequently allied "asthma." The author does report those cases in which it failed, and although he came to see it as the most efficacious agent for dropsy, he tried it occasionally in other disorders, such as consumption. It was probably not possible for him, within the eighteenth-century medical mindset, to conceive of a drug as more or less a "specific" for a particular disease. The categorization of diseases remained too elastic, while drugs were mostly thought of as influencing one or more general body processes, not reversing some very focal abnormality, much less eradicating a particular microbe or acting at some cell receptor. Nonetheless, through his observed and compiled clinical experience, Withering was able to offer guidance on which sort of dropsical persons would be most likely to benefit. He became familiar with the well-known adverse effects of digitalis, particularly gastric upset, excess slowing of the heart rate, and the peculiar distortions of color vision. He offered further advice on watching for these side effects as a way to gauge the amount and timing of doses—he tamed the foxglove. No ordinary country physician, Withering excelled as a botanist and held membership in the important scientific societies of his day. It is not surprising that he would seek general principles for the employment of the drug. His *Account of the Foxglove,* however, is a wholly practical text, with very little attempt to discuss how and why digitalis might work.

Into the twentieth century, digitalis became the preeminent drug for heart diseases. It is still in wide use for the treatment of edema and breathlessness when caused by heart failure, and for certain rhythm disorders of the heart, though newer drugs have reduced reliance on it. Toxic effects appear at doses of the drug only slightly above those that are therapeutic: it has always been a troublesome member of the *materia medica*. Two hundred years after Withering, it became possible to dose the drug much better by measuring levels of digitalis in the blood. Still, Withering's *Account of the Foxglove* represents what might be the first thorough and adequate analysis of the use of a particular drug, and digitalis itself stands as one of the few enduring pre-nineteenth-century medicines in Western practice. Withering and foxglove were important characters in the biography of dropsy.

TRAVELS AND TAPPINGS FOR DROPSY: THE EXPERIENCE OF HENRY FIELDING

More than occasionally, dropsy would not yield to any medication. Then, recourse might be had to more extreme measures. If a person could bear it, one such option was the trochar—the instrument used to tap through the abdominal wall and free the waters within. The other, if one could afford it, was a trip, perhaps over the water, to a warmer climate: doctors and knowledgeable patients knew that cold begets and sustains the dropsy. In 1753, at the age of forty-seven, the English playwright, novelist, and civil servant Henry Fielding (1707–1754) found himself in much reduced health—"a very weak and deplorable condition," as he called it, "with no fewer or less diseases than a jaundice, a dropsy, and an asthma, altogether uniting their forces in the destruction of a body so entirely emaciated that it had lost all its muscular flesh."[32] Drugs had failed him. As it happens, he pursued a cure with *both* tapping and travel, and wrote of this unusual compound therapy in his *Journal of a Voyage to Lisbon*. He wrote because he was a writer and because accounts of travel were popular at the time. Perhaps the words he placed on paper helped give some meaning, as well as usefulness, to his misery.

Dealing as magistrate with a series of murders and robberies had kept Fielding in London during a brutal winter. In February of 1754, he consulted a Dr. Ward (probably Joshua "Spot" Ward, considered by some a quack). "By his advice I was tapped, and fourteen quarts of water drawn from my belly. The sudden relaxation which this caused, added to my enervate, emaciated habit of body, so weakened me that within two days I was thought to be falling into the agonies of death." Fielding rallied, but so did the dropsy, so he underwent another tapping about two months later and "bore all the consequences of the operation much better," which he attributed to the surgeon (not Ward himself) having prescribed a dose of laudanum, an opiate. It being now early May but still chilly in London, Fielding resolved to visit "a little house of mine in the country," in Middlesex, which offered "the best air, I believe, in the whole kingdom."[33] "But, by the end of May," wrote the novelist, "my belly became again ripe for the trochar, and I was a third time tapped; upon which, two very favorable symptoms appeared. I had three quarts of water taken from me less than had been taken the last time; and I bore the relaxation with much less (indeed with scarce any) faintness."[34] May proved virtually sunless, and Fielding (with the dropsy yet again gaining ground) feared that summer would elude Britain altogether. "I now began to recall an intention, which from the first dawnings of my recovery I had conceived, of removing to a warmer climate; and, finding this to be approved of by a very eminent physician, I resolved to put it into immediate execution." He fixed on Lisbon, which "must be more mild and warm, and the winter shorter and less piercing," and booked passage on a ship.[35]

As the ship prepared to depart London in late June (following several delays), Fielding feared that the water would rise within him during the voyage, and found that the lad serving as ship's surgeon had never tapped for dropsy. "By way of prevention, therefore, I this day sent for my friend, Mr. Hunter, the great surgeon and anatomist of Covent-garden; and, though my belly was not yet very full and tight, let out ten quarts of water; the young sea-surgeon attending the operation, not as a performer, but as a student."[36] In late July, as the slow-moving ship was finally about to leave the south shores of England for Portugal, Fielding sent for a surgeon from a nearby town for another drainage. "I was now once more delivered from my burden. . . . While the surgeon was drawing away my water, the sailors were drawing up the anchor; both were finished at the same time; we unfurled our sails and soon passed the Berryhead, which forms the mouth of the bay."[37]

Fielding reached the warmer city of Lisbon, but the new setting could not cure his dropsy or other onerous diseases, and he died there two months later. We can note several aspects of Fielding's quest for relief, in addition to the pursuit of warmth. Like Samuel Johnson, as a man of education and some status, he knew something about dropsy and did not passively submit to treatment. He chose at one point to try the putative remedy "tar water" of which he had read, and himself scheduled his tappings. Though not wealthy, he could afford the practitioners he desired, and the journey south. After his first paracentesis, he suffered the general collapse that commonly follows removal of a large amount of fluid from the abdomen—recipients of the treatment often feel literally "drained," and this phenomenon is still seen when the operator takes off too much fluid at once. Andrew Jackson underwent a tapping for his dropsy, done in seeming desperation a few days before he died, and although he gained some relief, it "totally prostrated the poor man."[38] Fielding, however, survived his first procedure and found the subsequent tappings easily tolerable. Many other patients, in contrast, found application of the trochar and its initial aftermath agonizing and refused a second drainage.

As mentioned at the start of this chapter, paracentesis to drain ascitic fluid was known in antiquity and has been done ever since. The seventeenth-century British surgeon Richard Wiseman described the technique for "giving vent to the water" this way: "I went provided for the work, and the Patient resolved to undergo the Opening. Other Symptoms to encourage me I had none. The next morning, she having prepared her self, and being placed on that side she could best lie upon during the Evacuation, her Bracer being well fitted, I made the Perforation according to custom three fingers below the Navel on the upper side. The water spurted out forcibly whilst I passed in my taper-pointed *Cannula,* which fitting exactly, I let out about three pints of Water."[39] A "bracer" was a tight bandage around the abdomen to create pressure that would help the fluid to escape; "three fingers below the Navel" marked the time-honored landmark. Wiseman applied several types of bandaging after the procedure, and later taught the servants how to let out some fluid each day by way of the cannula.

Tapping the abdomen has long been a well-known event in the

life of the dropsical person. Fielding wrote as if his readers would readily know what he meant when he said, "I was tapped, and fourteen quarts of water drawn from my belly." So did George Eliot, describing a character tapped "no end o' times" in *The Mill on the Floss*. In fact, those who had undergone many insertions of the trochar and cannula sometimes obtained a sort of celebrity status in either the lay or popular press. The *Gentleman's Magazine* of London in its January 1732 issue told of the Widow Haggard of Shriverham "who had been tapp'd for the Dropsy 21 Times, [and] was ready to be tapp'd again." A table provided the dates and amounts (in gallons) for each evacuation.[40] The same publication in September of 1737 offered details of an elderly woman of Worcester who overall underwent fifty tappings and "had extracted from her in all 116 Gallons of Water."[41] Presumably, the gentlemen found these statistics somehow amusing.

A listing of "enormous dropsies" and individuals who were tapped immense numbers of times appears in Gould and Pyle's amazing *Anomalies and Curiosities of Medicine*, first published in 1897. Though aimed at the medical profession, "popular editions" of this illustrated and sensational work eventually appeared, and it remains available in online renditions.[42] Within twenty-first-century medicine, physicians still often carry out paracentesis to drain out ascitic fluid, particularly in the setting of cirrhosis of the liver. Indeed, the procedure has been subjected to that most current of interrogations, the controlled clinical trial, to see how it compares with other types of treatments.[43] Paracentesis can claim something like transcendent status in Western medicine. It has been a procedure in use almost throughout that medicine's recorded history, a therapeutic action that has ignored theory while it has visibly and irrefutably done the job.

⟨⟨⟨⟩⟩⟩

Dropsy, in its day, was no trifling sickness, even if it is now extinct as a "disease" in the present-day meaning. It caused awful suffering and changed the body in grotesque ways that altered the patient's sense of self. A soldier and president, the "man of iron will," saw himself, near the end of life, as a "blubber of water." It could deprive the body of life's breath and of life itself. The suffering could persuade patients to ingest all manner of noisome drugs, including foxglove, or digitalis, but it was dropsy that taught William Withering how to tame this valuable medicinal for heart disease. Withering and his book attained permanent fame. Patients also consented to, or even requested, paracentesis and tolerated feeling their abdomens punctured by a quite sizeable needle, sometimes dozens of times over months or years. A few such individuals gained unwanted commemoration as record-challenging subjects of repeated tappings for dropsy. Others found the first attempt or its immediate consequences terrifying and preferred to die rather than undergo the operation a second time.

As with any serious illness, dropsy possessed a certain social authority. Obviously, when severe enough, it removed and excused the victim from the usual responsibilities of life and placed her or him in the chair, to be cared for, or at least visited, if there were family or friends to do so. As we have seen, it could occasionally display the power to send someone on a sea voyage, to a warmer climate less conducive to the "cold," phlegmatic swelling. For elite physicians, dropsy could supply opportunities for something like research (Withering), and for the writing of books that could both share observations and therapeutic advice, and perhaps elevate one's standing within the profession. Surgeons could display the virtues of their practical approach to the sick: the trochar and cannula go in, the fluid comes out, and who will really care whether it was a cold humor or some problem of the "exhaling system" that caused the mischief.

The dropsical sufferers we have presented—Johnson, Fielding, briefly Jackson—became dropsical, received treatment, and died dropsical in their house, not in a hospital. They were, of course, persons of some means, who would not have resorted to a hospital when sick. Before the late nineteenth century, nothing could be done there diagnostically or therapeutically that could not be done at home, and hospitals were dangerous places. Those in the beds might die of whatever ailment placed them there, or of some fever caught within the walls. The indigent and the working poor took refuge in hospitals when no other option for care existed. In the next chapter, we shift focus to the "hospital medicine" of the early nineteenth century and an outgrowth of it—the remapping of disease through correlation of the clinical signs with the findings at autopsy. In this new medical environment, disease still wielded power and patients still claimed the capacity to accept or refute a doctor's recommendation; but physicians gained new sources of authority. With the new clinical-pathological methods, physicians and surgeons assumed the right to dismiss old diseases and propose new ones. Dropsy, something everyone easily recognized and knew how to deal with since the age of Hippocrates, somehow evaporated as a useful, or usable, denomination of disease. Partly in its place appeared a malady with a novel sort of name and a novel means of diagnosis—Bright's Disease.

—⟳⟳⟳—

A Later Perspective

As mentioned, dropsy is now a largely archaic term within medicine. There are two exceptions. "Epidemic dropsy" is a toxigenic disorder seen in India, caused by adulterated mustard seed oil. An affliction of aquarium fish, marked by a swollen belly, still goes by the name "dropsy." In current medicine, "ascites" still refers to fluid in the abdominal cavity, "edema" to fluid within tissues elsewhere (especially the legs), and "anasarca" to an extreme degree of fluid overload throughout the body, the sum of widespread edema and ascites. All of these result from an imbalance of salt (sodium and chloride) and water management in the body, mediated by the failure of the kidneys to discharge enough salt and water through urine. Retention of salt (failure of excretion of salt by the kidneys) is as important as, or more important than, that of water, because water "follows" salt. More on this below. In general, edema and ascites (for brevity, I'll use the general term "edema" from here on) occur as consequences of certain diseases of the heart, liver, and, of course, the kidneys. How does this happen?

Each human kidney comprises about one million units called nephrons, each of which consists of a microscopic ball of blood capillaries called the glomerulus, and a twisting tubular structure called, not surprisingly, the renal tubule. The glomerulus is a sieve, or filter, through which blood passes, and the filtrate it separates from the blood passes down the tubule. There, most of the salt and water that had been removed from the blood are reabsorbed (drawn back) into the minute blood vessels surrounding the tubule in such a way that the final urine—the sum product of all the nephrons of both kidneys—normally contains the metabolic wastes needing removal from the body, and exactly the right amount of salt and water that need to be ejected. Substances that the body ought not lose in the urine, such as sugar and amino acids—the building blocks of proteins—are also reabsorbed by the tubules and retained. These essential substances are reabsorbed mainly by the part of the tubule just following the glomerulus, called the "proximal tubule." Regulatory systems adjust the reabsorption processes by the kidney to maintain the physiologically correct content of salt and water in the body. These systems involve hormones, or messenger substances, such as aldosterone (which induces the kidney tubule to save sodium) and vasopressin (also called antidiuretic hormone), which urges the tubule to save water. The fine adjustments of exactly how much water and salt to retain, versus how much to discharge into the final urine, are handled mainly by the last parts of the tubule, called the distal tubule and collecting duct.

Salt (sodium with its chloride and bicarbonate anions) is the dominant chemical constituent of the blood plasma, the fluid part of the blood, which conveys the red and white cells and essential nutrients throughout the body. As a legacy of some fishlike origins of mammals, it is the amount of salt in the blood plasma that determines the volume, or amount, of the plasma and thus of the ability of blood to achieve the circulation of oxygen-carrying red cells, nutrients, and so on. Thus, if the blood plasma volume becomes low, certain sensors trigger a message to the kidneys' tubules to retain (reabsorb) salt, and water follows the salt through something known as "osmotic force." In heart failure, the inability of the cardiac pump to propel the blood forward through the arterial system more or less "fools" the sensors into reading a low volume. This false reading eventually causes the kidneys to retain salt, and with it water, in an attempt to increase blood volume. But, in heart failure, the volume is not truly deficient, so the exaggerated retention of salt and water overfills the circulation (the system of moving blood in arteries and veins). Some of the salt and water oozes out of the overfilled blood, into surrounding tissues (known as the "interstitium," in effect the elastic areas mostly surrounding muscles) and into the abdominal cavity. This is the dropsy, or edema. Similar

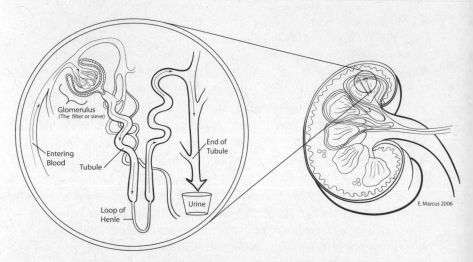

Schematic drawing of a nephron unit, showing glomerulus and tubule. Drawn for the author by Elisheva Marcus.

movement of salt and water out of the overfilled bloodstream into the lungs causes the breathlessness of heart failure.

Something similar, but more complex and less well understood, occurs with cirrhosis of the liver, another disease associated with edema and ascites—and no doubt a longtime source of the idea that dropsy is linked to jaundice and the liver, and with alcoholism. In a cirrhotic person, an intense and counterproductive signal to the kidneys causes them to vastly overretain salt and water.

Of course, kidney disease itself can cause edema and ascites, and commonly does. If any acute or chronic disorder of the kidneys has destroyed most of the nephron units, or somehow impaired their function, a person will gain bodily salt and water if the maximum amount that the injured kidneys can discharge each day does not match the amounts ingested (some water will also be lost across the skin and through the lungs). When the particular form of renal disease causes a large loss of blood protein through the kidneys (as will be discussed in chapter 2), lowering the content of protein (especially albumin) in the blood, a process known as nephrotic syndrome can emerge. It is associated with a distinct tendency for the renal tubules to reabsorb sodium, leading to edema as water follows the salt.

Modern drugs known as diuretics or "water pills" work by partly blocking some of the salt (sodium) reabsorption by the renal tubules: as more salt is thereby allowed to flow out in the urine, more water goes out as well. The salt and water thereby removed from the blood plasma are replenished from the burden of excess salt and water—the edema—in the tissues of the legs and in the abdomen. Such agents (the most widely known in the United States are furosemide and a class of diuretics known as the thiazides) can be very effective in reducing edema, though they do not directly influence the underlying disease of the heart, liver, or kidneys. It is not known to what extent the drugs of earlier times that were considered diuretic actually owned such properties. As pointed out earlier, however, even the loss from the body of salt and water through the use of laxatives and emetics can be expected to gradually reduce the body's excess stores of salt and water and therefore improve the symptom of edema. Withering and those who followed long believed that digitalis (foxglove) acted as a diuretic, and to some degree such might be the case. But its main effect is now understood to be on the heart, where it can make regular an erratic rhythm of the heartbeat and also improve the pumping strength of the organ. Thus it is most effective, and sometimes dramatically so, in treating edema when administered to the patient with heart failure. Yet it seemed to work in some of Withering's patients who, as best one can tell, probably did not have cardiac disease.

In patients with severe loss of kidney function, even the most powerful diuretics will not work, because there simply remain too few nephron units to excrete salt, water, or anything else. In such a situation, edema amounts to only one of the manifestations of the renal disease, and all can be treated with temporary or permanent replacement of kidney function by hemodialysis, the "artificial kidney." This treatment, of course, will be addressed later in this book.

CHAPTER TWO

Richard Bright's New Disease

❧

Chapter 1 contains the illness narratives of two men of letters, but neither medical training nor high education was needed to recognize dropsy and to know something about it. Rural clergyman and farmer Ralph Josselin easily diagnosed it in himself in 1683, a contributor to the *Gentleman's Magazine* provided an ode to mark his recovery from the disorder in 1751, and the country ladies in *The Mill on the Floss* chatted casually about the notable case of dropsy in their parish.[1] Dropsy was disease as very visible symptom. The malady called Bright's Disease, on the other hand, arose from the invisible made visible. The nineteenth-century English physician Richard Bright (1789–1858) proved something new about dropsy, something previously only hinted at here and there, and ignored. By regularly carrying out autopsies when dropsical patients died, Bright found that in some cases the kidneys showed striking distortions in their structure. Some were swollen and bloody red, others smooth and pale, many smallish, hard, and "granulated." Dropsy accompanied by pathological alterations in the kidneys, and by albuminous urine (more on this later in the chapter), came to be known as Bright's Disease, Bright's Kidney, or the morbus Brightii (none of these were names Bright chose). He published his discovery initially in a large, handsomely produced illustrated book. Let us look carefully at one illustration from that book, Bright's *Reports of Medical Cases* of 1827.[2]

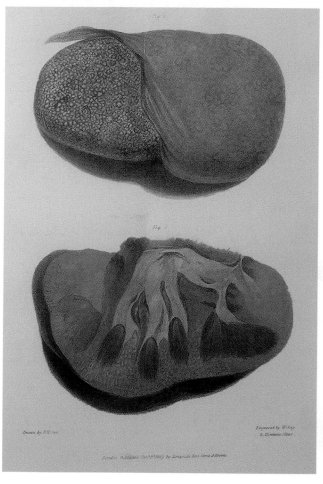

"Kidney in Dropsy," plate 1 from vol. 1 of Richard Bright's *Reports of Medical Cases* of 1827. This is the "granulated kidney" indicative of long-standing disease. Courtesy of the Library of the College of Physicians of Philadelphia.

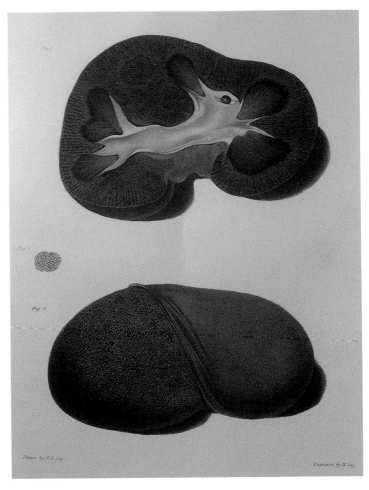

"Kidney in Dropsy," plate 5 from vol. 1 of Richard Bright's *Reports of Medical Cases* of 1827. The appearance suggests what later became known as acute glomerulonephritis, a disease sometimes related to streptococcal infection of the throat or skin. Courtesy of the Library of the College of Physicians of Philadelphia.

The image of the dropsical woman in chapter 1 showed a patient, and a very complete patient: no one can fail to see her dropsical symptoms, part of her treatment, and her abysmal misery. Although Bright's magnificent book is full of detailed patient stories, its illustrations show only diseased *organs*—particularly kidneys, livers, lungs, and brains. The first plate in the book is labeled on its opposite page "Kidney in Dropsy." We are told that the upper figure shows "one of the kidneys of King, from half of which the tunic is removed, showing an advanced stage of that granulated condition of the organ which was in this case connected with the secretion of albuminous urine.—Anasarca and hydrothorax [fluid in the chest cavity] accompanied this disease." The bottom figure is a "longitudinal section of the same kidney, showing the most advanced stage of the granular change."

The upper figure reveals to the left the surface of the kidney. Ordinarily, it would be smooth and pink. But here we see a kind of pimply, granulated appearance, with spots of red, yellow, and other colors. The tunic (or what today is called the capsule, a fibrous sheathing of the kidney) has been snipped away; Bright (who did most of the autopsies himself) had entered the darkness of the interior of the body, then further penetrated to unwrap the kidney, seeking to find the hidden "seat" of the illness. Then, the kidney has been sliced to gain further visualization of its internal appearance, which merely confirms the "granular change" and some loss of the normal landmarks that would be familiar to the experienced anatomist. The kidneys are printed life-size, and the illustrator has attempted to convey three-dimensionality through customary uses of shading. He has even indicated how the kidneys throw down a shadow—a touch that is entirely unneeded for the purpose, but to show the shadow no doubt was second nature to the experienced artist, and to do it properly, a mark of competence. The shadow conveys that this was a real kidney, a piece of the body, with mass and weight. Yet the shadow seems to fall on nothing—there is no pan, or board, on which the kidney sits, and certainly it has not been portrayed in situ, in the corpse of the patient, Mr. King. It is the actual diseased kidney of a particular sick individual, removed from the body, presented full-size, in color, free of distractions —and if not glorified, at least invested with decisive importance.

A much later critique of medicine has seen Bright's time as the era when patients became "objectified"—thought of by physicians mainly in terms of their deranged organs—"the cirrhotic liver in bed twelve" or "the granular kidney in bed fifteen." No doubt such was an approaching trend in medicine, as it became transformed by the "localist" pathology of the early nineteenth century, particularly in France. Certainly Richard Bright of London partook in the fascination for finding the "seat" of the illness at autopsy and in minutely examining the disembodied organ. But he seems to have been as well a humane physician. One biographer, with access to family letters, reports that Bright "watched over" one favorite patient, even hand-fed him some food and wine, "holding his wrist till the end."[3] A former pupil at Guy's Hospital recalled Bright as "kindness itself to the poor patients under his charge."[4] When Bright published his initial cases of albuminous renal disease, he included each patient's name and occupation—"sailor," "carpenter," "needle-work," "drover," and so on. Certainly Bright's private patients were "persons" to him, not just diseases, and these included friends and family members. But for Bright the "medical scientist," to permit myself another anachronistic term, it was knowledge about the diseased organs that offered the promise of progress in medicine. And he went to substantial trouble to show his readers such organs.

Although not easily seen in our reproduction, at the bottom of the original page one discerns to the left the words "Drawn by F. R. Say," and to the right, "Engraved by W. Say, 9 Mortimer Street." Frederick Richard Say (1805–1860) counted among the popular portrait painters of London, and his father William Say (1768–1834) was a skilled engraver active in the ornamental print market. The elder Say practiced the craft of mezzotint engraving, a technique that avoided the stereotypic cross-hatching associated with the common copperplate process. Mezzotint could yield striking and lovely effects in suggesting volume and in portraying the texture of surfaces. This suited Bright's need—to show the grainy surface of the diseased kidneys. Of the forty illustrative plates in the entire *Reports of Medical Cases,* five (all by the Says) show variants of the kidney changes associated with dropsy and albuminous urine.

Bright, the author and manager of the large book, believed that the illustrations were critical, perhaps decisive, in proving his case for a "new" disease that would become, literally, *his* new disease once the name "Bright's Disease" became fixed in usage. Pathology above all was a visual science and practice. Bright no doubt wanted the illustrations to convey to the reader's eyes the detail that he saw at the time of autopsy and to give credibility to the discoveries, very much as a photograph might do once that invention found its use in science. So he undertook a time-consuming and costly process. He had to engage an established painter (the younger Say) to appear at the Guy's Hospital morgue to render a color painting of a fresh specimen. Later, the elder Say, using the painting as a model, would at leisure produce the mezzotint plate to be used for making the final prints.

The engraving process leads to a black-and-white image, but the original *colors* of the diseased organ demanded reproduction. Physicians had long relied on color in making a diagnosis. They attended to the pallor of consumption or anemia, the redness of inflammation, the yellowing of skin with liver disease, the greenness of that mysteriously extinct malady called chlorosis. Even the old humoral system balanced red, black, yellow, and white. In turn, nineteenth-century pathologists depended upon color as well in analyzing and classifying the alterations they would identify in organs and tissues of the body, and eventually (using stains), in preparations viewed through the microscope. Well outside of medicine, artists such as Englishman J. M. W. Turner romantically and gorgeously spread color in their paintings in new ways. But no simple process for printing in color existed in the 1820s and 1830s. For each of the several hundred copies of the *Reports of Medical Cases* produced, each illustration was skillfully hand-colored with water paints, presumably using the original painting as a guide. Yet, examination of two copies of the plates side by side, with a magnifying lens, reveals almost no discrepancy. Precisely how the coloring—which in many plates remains gloriously vivid—was accomplished may never be known.

What is clear is that the process, which Dr. Bright paid for himself, limited the "press run" of the *Reports of Medical Cases* and made it very costly.[5] But the book was purchased and read, as were similar treatises and colored atlases, mainly from France and Great Britain, that advanced the knowledge and authority of pathology. At this time, "pathology" meant the quest for the center, or focus, of disease in some particular place or places within the body, an organ or set of organs changed in some recognizable and definable manner. Colored plates enhanced the credibility of claims made by pathologists and at least theoretically made it possible for a physician-pathologist doing an autopsy in Dublin to recognize a species of pathological abnormality documented in Vienna.[6] Speculating about which humor caused the dropsy, or accepting it as the "watery-cold" distemper, no longer would suffice in the vibrant new medical world of the 1820s, where disease was being remapped through the colors and textures of pathology.

RICHARD BRIGHT AND THE SETTING OF HIS WORK

We may recall from chapter 1 that the celebrated Samuel Johnson, having died dropsical, received an autopsy that uncovered pathological changes in the heart and kidneys. Some readers might think that persons of some means and reputation would have escaped postmortem examination in 1784, but in fact, dissecting dead bodies had become common practice. Dissection of the human body occurred, it is believed, in the classical world, then disappeared within the Christian and Moslem nations of the early Middle Ages. It was revived in the European universities in the fourteenth and fifteenth centuries and became a passionate pursuit of medical anatomists and several artists of the Renaissance. Andreas Vesalius (1514–1564), Belgian born but working in Padua, became the leading figure in the rebirth of anatomy. His magisterial *De Humani Corporis Fabrica* (*On the Structure of the Human Body*) of 1543, with its well-known woodcut illustrations, described the body in detail never before seen, and corrected several errors long perpetuated from the anatomy of the ancient authority Galen, which was largely based on animals. The objective of Vesalius, Leonardo, and many others who dissected during the Renaissance was to understand the normal structure of the human being—as a study for its own sake and to better understand the Divine fabricator.

Beginning at no identifiable date, and with no single impetus, once a fairly good grasp of normal anatomy had been attained, physicians next took interest in variations from normal as revealed by autopsy. They saw and described organs swollen, shrunken, ulcerated, altered in color or texture—enwrapping membranes thickened, thinned, weeping, or studded with tubercles. And much more. British physician and anatomist William Harvey (1578–1657), working (like Vesalius) in Padua, is celebrated for his brilliant description of the workings of the heart and circulation, published as *De Motu Cordis* in 1628. He also studied "morbid" (diseased) anatomy, though on this he never published. In 1761, Giovanni Battista Morgagni (1682–1771) of Padua (Padua was a center of anatomical study) in 1761 published his enormous *De Sedibus, et Causis Morborum per Anatomen Indagatis* (*On the Sites and Causes of Disease, Indicated by Anatomy*), a systematic compilation of about seven hundred autopsies done by him or others. This massive work attempted to link the clinical symptoms in the living person with findings on postmortem examination. This would become the central objective: remap the domain of diseases by lining up the pattern of symptoms with the underlying disordered structure. To this end, the Scot Matthew Baillie (1761–1823) offered one of the earliest English-language treatises on pathology in 1793, *The Morbid Anatomy of Some of the Most Important Parts of the Human Body,* which, accompanied eventually by an atlas of illustrations, underwent numerous reprints and new editions.[7]

But it was postrevolutionary France that became the unquestioned seat and center of a widespread "programmatic" effort by physician-pathologists to replace the long serviceable classification of diseases based on *symptoms,* with one built upon *structural change in organs or tissues.* This program also included attempts to better categorize and understand the processes, or mechanisms, of disease. Why did France, and especially Paris, become the locus for this early nineteenth-century program, which history has long associated with the names of Xavier Bichat, R. T. H. Laennec, Pierre Louis, Pierre-Joseph Desault, and others? Several reasons can be offered. First, the revolutionary spirit favored skepticism concerning old ways of thinking and practicing. Second, the new program to correlate patterns of symptoms in the living, with internal findings at autopsy, more or less demanded the *hospital set-*

ting: in the hospital, large numbers of the sick, many suffering the gravest forms of illness, are gathered together, and many will die. The sheer numbers allow for the discovery of repeated patterns. Hospitals for the working poor and the indigent existed well before 1800 in the major cities of Europe. However, they proliferated particularly in Paris, where the postrevolutionary "rationalized" arrangements made the patients, living or dead, available for study by what we would now call academic physicians carrying out research. Finally, the postrevolutionary reform of medical education brought the training of surgeons and physicians together, allowing the "localist" eye and mind of the surgeon to influence the thinking of the medical men.[8]

A "tradition" of clinical-pathological correlation, however, existed in Britain too, as we've pointed out, and it is not surprising that British clinicians of the early decades of the nineteenth century who were attracted to this sort of work read the publications of the leading French workers and sometimes went to study with them. Such an ambitious Englishman was Richard Bright, who was born in Bristol to an affluent family of bankers and merchant-venturers but spent his medical career mainly in London.[9] He could allow himself a lengthy period of medical training, which comprised clinical tutelage on the wards of Guy's Hospital, lectures and examinations at the University of Edinburgh leading to its medical degree in 1813, then several years of hard work at London dispensaries and at a "fever hospital." Following this preparation, he opened a private practice and received appointment as a staff physician at Guy's Hospital, "the largest repository of disease in the metropolis" and a prominent site of medical education in association with nearby St. Thomas's Hospital. A staff surgeon, Astley Cooper, cast a strong influence on the United Hospitals (as the affiliation was known). The surgeon's desire has always been to find the patient's trouble within the space of the body, to visualize it, and to treat it locally. Richard Bright long had been fond of the visual. As a child, he acquired proficiency in geology, a pastime of his father, and as a young man showed unusual skill in drawing and sketching. He could "think" visually, was alert to color, and had become an astute observer.

Many physicians of Bright's time (and other professional persons) cultivated "natural history," the descriptive study of nature, including classification and illustration. For Bright, one might think of his work in pathology as extending the love of natural history to medicine. Although he would eventually have a lot of mouths to feed (seven children who survived infancy), his family's wealth had permitted a long period of self-directed medical training and travel, including, briefly, to Paris. The same affluence at least partly freed Bright from the need to build a large "business." He could therefore devote time to his chosen work—pathology and clinical-pathological correlation. As a doctor, he took care of all sorts of people and observed the entire spectrum of diseases. But Bright took special interest in dropsy, of which there was no shortage among the ailing occupants of Guy's Hospital.

INTRODUCING BRIGHT'S DISEASE

Several physicians before Bright knew that certain individuals with dropsy showed a curious abnormality in their urine: if a bit of it was heated, by placing some in a spoon over a lighted candle, a coagulum formed, which seemed in appearance identical to heated egg albumin. William Charles Wells (1757–1817) and John Blackall (1771–1860), both British practitioners (Wells was American born), even had found that a few such patients when coming to autopsy showed abnormalities of the kidneys, among other findings, but they did not fully perceive a relationship. At some point in the early 1820s, Bright began performing this simple (and one might now say "cost-effective") test on the urine of his dropsical patients—or he had one of his pupils do it. He ensured that careful notes were maintained describing the clinical symptoms and course of the patients, which of them had "coagulable" urine, and the treatments administered. Many of these ill people died and received postmortem dissection—the *sectio cadaveris*. Bright's contribution was to declare, with sufficient numbers to convince, this fact: those dropsical patients who had coagulable urine, and not the others, would show one or another form of structurally altered kidney at the postmortem examination. "I have never yet examined the body of a patient dying with dropsy attended with coagulable urine, in whom some obvious derangement was not discovered in the kidneys."[10] Bright's Disease initially, then, amounted to a triad: dropsy, the symptom that the person experienced; coagulable urine (albumin in the urine), a "laboratory finding" in later terms; and "deranged" kidneys, the underlying pathology, revealed at autopsy.

But Bright and colleagues soon became aware that there was sometimes more to it than this. Some of the dropsical patients with albuminuria displayed other symptoms, all throughout their bodies, sometimes hectic and horrific. John King, the intemperate sailor introduced above, developed intense shortness of breath and "inflammation in the chest." When Bright listened with his stethoscope (still a novelty in 1825), the sounds of the heartbeat seemed quiet, "as if performed through fluid."[11] The autopsy showed an inflamed pericardium (the fibrous wrapping of the heart) and fluid trapped between the pericardium and heart.

The thirteenth case of the *Reports of Medical Cases,* Thomas Drudget, was a carman, "by no means an intemperate man . . . always passing the evenings with his family."[12] Not dropsy, but vomiting had marked the beginning of his illness, though he soon swelled up. Two weeks after his admission to Guy's, the end of his illness, and of his life, came with violent seizures. The autopsy showed, in addition to diseased kidneys, a hemorrhage into the brain. Bright also had noted that Drudget's pulse was "sharp with a jerk," not uncommon among the dropsical-albuminous patients.[13]

By the time of publication of the first volume of the *Reports,* in 1827, Bright concluded that the inflammation of the "serous" and mucous membranes of the body commonly arose in these dropsical patients with underlying kidney disease. By "serous" membranes, he referred to the pericardium, to the pleural linings of the lung, and to the peritoneal linings of the abdominal cavity. He also warned that the brain often participated in the overall illness, since both "apoplexy and epilepsy" were seen to occur in some cases ("apoplexy" meant something like "stroke").[14]

With a large enough number of people available to observe, record, and think about, Bright was able to extend and confirm his perception of a "pattern," what later might be considered a "syndrome," a recognizable set or complex of disease manifestations. The syndrome that he was assembling eventually became known as uremia, the set of symptoms and findings that accompany overall reduction of the kidneys' excretory ability and that is presumably caused by some retained toxic substances. By the time of his second major publication on renal disease, in 1836, Bright had worked out a more or less "fixed" or recognizable "history of this disease, and its symptoms."[15] Also by this time, he had encountered cases less severe than those detailed in the *Reports of Medical Cases* and grasped that a more "chronic" form of the disorder existed, characterized by a fitful pattern of exacerbations and remissions. Among the common elements of albuminous kidney disease, in addition to dropsy, Bright included: the "pulse full and hard"; headache; dry skin; a fading of "the healthy colour of the countenance"; vomiting; and "a sense of lassitude, of weariness, and of depression" that "steal over the bodily and mental frame." The clinical course shows ups and downs: "The swelling increases and decreases; the mind grows cheerful or is sad; the secretions of the kidney or skin are augmented or diminished." The person may rally and "enters on his active duties," but he may at any time see a return of the old symptoms or suffer an attack of pericarditis, or of peritonitis. A sudden convulsion, or a sinking into coma, marks the end of the struggle.

THE NAME "BRIGHT'S DISEASE"

Although Richard Bright did not propose the name, the disease or diseases he described quickly became known as morbus Brightii, Bright's Kidney, maladie de Bright in French, or most commonly, Bright's Disease. "Bright's Disease" may be the earliest regularly used eponymous name for a disease in English, that is, a disease named for its "discoverer" (in a different sense, of course, it was the patients who first knew about it).[16] It is the only such disease name in the index to the 1844 edition of Thomas Watson's popular *Lectures on the Principles and Practice of Physic,* a standard medical text of its day. Watson, however, did not like the term. "For this disease," he wrote, "we have no appropriate name. I wish we had. Some call it *granular degeneration* of the kidney, but the epithet granular is not always applicable. It is most familiarly known, both here and abroad, as *Bright's kidney,* or *Bright's disease;* after the eminent physician who in 1837 [*sic*; should be 1827] first described it, and showed its great pathological importance. These are odd-sounding and awkward terms; but in the lack of better, I must employ them."[17] Other medical authors also disliked the name or found it peculiar.

Why did the naming of this new disease pose a problem and lead to a new way of naming diseases? Bright's Disease required a new sort of naming because it represented a new way of thinking about and defining disease, which had not existed before the early nineteenth century. Someone had Bright's Disease if he had at least some of the following: certain symptoms, such as dropsy; certain physical findings, such as a "sharp pulse," or a frictional, rubbing sound heard over the heart using the stethoscope; certain morbid changes in the kidney, if he came to autopsy; and—perhaps most novel in the 1820s and 1830s—an early sort of laboratory abnormality, albuminous urine. Several of these elements—albuminuria, cardiac "rub" heard through the stethoscope, morbid changes of the kidney—*only the physician could detect*. So this sickness is no longer only the ill person's disease: it's also the physician's disease, Dr. Bright's disease.

Bright's Disease, and other "new" diseases that would be defined by the stethoscope, the laboratory, or the autopsy, represented a shift in the structure of medicine itself and in the patient-doctor relationship. Of course physicians had long exercised the function of declaring a diagnosis, though for such "diseases" as dropsy, fever, hemorrhage, or consumption, it would be all too obvious to the sufferer. But with disease entities such as Bright's, much more authority rested with physicians or "medical science." Indeed, into the later nineteenth century, a physician might (rightly or wrongly) diagnose Bright's Disease in a person with only the most vague or minor symptoms—or none at all—if a urine examination happened to show a trace of albuminuria, which in small amounts causes no complaints. This represented an entirely new manner of transforming a person into a patient, and a new jurisdiction of medicine. The felt bodily sensations of the patient, and the patient's recounted story of them, would increasingly lose their primacy and power. Eventually, countless persons would find themselves, through measurement devices, assigned diseases that usually lacked symptoms: essential hypertension, or hyperlipidemia, and eventually—as will be seen in chapter 9—"chronic kidney disease" as designated by a single mildly abnormal blood test called creatinine.

This modern sort of diagnosis of the well would have been entirely mysterious to Richard Bright, but he did come to recognize that not all the components of his new disease were always present. For example, case five reported in his 1836 article "Cases and Observations Illustrative of Renal Disease Accompanied with the Secretion of Albuminous Urine" provides "a strong example of the disease of the kidney passing to its most fatal period, without the slightest symptom of dropsical effusion—a state of things, which, above all, is apt to throw us off our guard."[18] Gradually it would become clear as well that some patients might progress to complete failure of the kidneys without ever showing important albuminuria. Others might display profound anasarca and albuminuria although their kidneys show no defect to the naked eye. This variability also favored the abstract name "Bright's Disease," since in at least some cases such alternative labels as "granular kidney" or "albuminous nephritis" could not apply. It was a term presumably useful, even indispensable, to most physicians until (as we will see later) about the 1930s and 1940s. It was a term that gradually became comprehensible and useful to patients. A simple and accessible name, "Bright's Disease" broadly referred to an ailment sufficiently common that many persons would have known, or known of, someone who had it. It probably meant to nonphysicians a way of getting sick through your kidneys, and that acquired a reputation for being a dangerous thing.

Indeed, as the nineteenth century progressed, Bright's Disease became known mainly as a chronic but incurable disorder. In 1878 the mother of a woman ill with fatigue and indistinct symptoms wrote to her son that "the Doctor frightened us out of our wits by suggesting Bright's disease of the kidney" as the diagnosis. The unwell woman was Lydia Cassatt, sister of the painter Mary Cassatt.[19] When the twenty-first American president, Chester Alan Arthur, was diagnosed with Bright's Disease in 1882, the popular understanding of this disorder demanded an official denial—"pure fiction."[20] Daniel W. Cathell, in his notorious but popular guide for new doctors called *The Physician Himself,* in 1882 listed

Bright's Disease along with tuberculosis and cancer as diagnoses that could extinguish all hope and interest in life if spoken too frankly.[21] (Actually, the spectrum of albuminuric kidney disease includes many cases that are indolent and unthreatening; maybe it acquired so fierce a reputation in the nineteenth century because it was first described through dissection of the dead and because the most serious cases would be most readily diagnosed.) As diagnostic labels often do, "Bright's Disease" had meaning beyond the descriptive or purely clinical: the name itself could raise terror and change one's life before it took one's life.

Like dropsy, Bright's Disease had the power to confine a person to home or set her traveling; to change her diet and change her dress. Lydia Cassatt, living with her sister in Paris, accepted a bland diet, and when her condition worsened, traveled to the warmer south of France on doctors' recommendations.[22] Bright's Disease, like other weighty diagnoses, certainly possessed that awful power to move a person from the realm of the "well" to that of the "no longer well," with all the consequences of that shift.[23] A person with arthritis of one or two joints, or some affliction of the eyes or ears, may still perceive himself or herself as well. But such a sense eludes those afflicted with symptomatic kidney disease, who deal with perturbations of the most essential functions of living—fatigue and inability to work, loss of appetite and failure to enjoy food, restlessness at night and interrupted sleep. All of these cause individual distress, and all erode customary social relationships of every sort. (We will encounter the experiences of others who suffered from Bright's Disease in chapter 3.)

THE HOUSE DISEASE OF GUY'S HOSPITAL

Bright's Disease quickly achieved another sort of power—it altered the organization of a hospital and its medical school, and provided something like a research agenda for its medical staff. In 1825, a dispute over the appointment of the lecturer in surgery brought to an end the joint medical school conducted by Guy's and nearby St. Thomas's Hospital. Under the forceful leadership of the "Treasurer" (really the senior managing officer) Benjamin Harrison, Guy's undertook to carry on an independent medical school.[24] (In this period, and long beyond it, medical schools in

Great Britain might be established by a hospital rather than a university, as would become the rule later, especially in the United States.) The initiation of Guy's separate medical school marked the beginning of a period of growth and reform at the institution, in which nepotism would be discouraged, the old system of selling the right to lecture (and presumably to pocket student fees) abolished, and an openness to newer ideas and research encouraged.

Treasurer Harrison was dictatorial but effective and in many ways progressive. He and his medical and surgical staff saw themselves now as rivals to their former partner, St. Thomas's, which had snubbed the Guy's choice for chief of surgery; they wanted to succeed and make a name for the new school. As some young British physicians, like Bright and his Guy's colleague Thomas Hodgkin, returned from long or short visits to Paris, they brought back a taste for producing and announcing new knowledge, particularly within pathology. An enlarging interest and expertise in medical chemistry among the British was largely homegrown. This was the setting of a hospital and medical school where Richard Bright introduced a new disease with multifaceted features, and in this setting, medical science at Guy's grew largely on the framework of Bright's Disease.

Though knowledgeable in geology and botany from a young age, Richard Bright apparently lacked facility in chemistry but recognized that the business of the kidney is chemical. Every physician knew the organs to be the "great depurators," the filters of the body, and that urine was a complex admixture of dissolved and half-dissolved chemical substances, as well as some particulate matter. Bright certainly did not look upon the spoon and candle test for urine coagulability as "chemistry" but seems in his descriptions of the various sorts of scum that might form to have seen it more as an extension of the physical examination of the patient. Nonetheless, he recognized that a full elaboration of kidney disease ought to include some chemical study. Just at the time he was identifying his albuminuric dropsical patients in the 1820s and 1830s, a "school" of clinical chemistry—chemistry applied to the problems of disease—was precociously making itself known in Britain.[25] It included physician-chemists William Prout, Alexander Marcet, George Owen Rees, Henry Bence Jones, and J. L. W.

Thudichum. When both were pupils at Guy's, Bright met Prout, later a leading practical chemist and theorist as well as practitioner. As mentioned in the *Reports,* Bright sent Prout several samples of urine and blood from the early renal patients for study, and Prout was able to tentatively conclude that the blood of one contained "a substance slightly analogous to urea." Blood always contains some urea, the waste product of protein metabolism in mammals, but Prout and Bright's other chemical collaborators were no doubt detecting elevated amounts with their crude techniques. It was urea that (as they surmised) the injured kidneys had failed to discharge. They knew that urea was a substance that the body needed to eliminate and that the kidneys took care of this.

Bright next turned to John Bostock, another physician with an interest in chemistry (among many other pursuits) and lecturer on chemistry at Guy's. He was able to show that the blood of several of the patients contained "less albumin than in health" and also thought he had found elevation of urea in blood.[26] Two Guy's pupils who would become staff members, Golding Bird and George Owen Rees, also tried their hand at looking for urea in the blood of patients with renal dropsy. Their differing findings and interpretations appeared for anyone to read as a series of contentious articles in a medical journal of the time.

During the 1830s, many pupils passing through Guy's busied themselves with small research projects dealing with kidney disease. The hospital had grown to five hundred beds, so there were lots of patients, dropsical and otherwise, lying about. Several students, outfitted with spoon and candle, set out to learn what proportion of all the bed patients showed albuminuria. Another of the illustrious physicians and teachers at Guy's, Thomas Addison, in 1839 published a paper on the neurological symptoms of Bright's Disease (Addison would eventually have a disease named for him—adrenal insufficiency). George H. Barlow, also a Guy's physician, described his use of "tartar emetic" (an antimonial medication) in acute cases of renal disorder. We have already noted that Thomas Hodgkin, the most French-influenced and skilled in pathology of the Guy's group, carried out some autopsies when Bright could not. (Hodgkin, of course, also acquired a pathological legacy, and "Hodgkin's Disease" to this day denotes a form of lymphatic cancer.) In 1836, Guy's launched its own journal, the *Guy's Hospital Reports*, to publish the research as well as therapeutic ideas emerging from the hospital and its school of medicine, particularly concerning kidney disease but of course also dealing with many other disorders. This step added to the prestige and standing Guy's desired within the world of British medicine.

In 1842 came the culmination of the institutional investigation of the new disease. Bright obtained permission from the management of Guy's to assign the two "clinical wards"—Job Ward and Lydia Ward, comprising the forty-two "teaching beds" used for "interesting" cases—entirely to the study of kidney disease from May through September. This was when bedside instruction was largely suspended. He considered it "the first experiment, which, as far as I know, has yet been made in this country to turn the ample resources of an hospital to the investigation of a particular disease, by bringing the patients labouring under it into one ward, properly arranged for observation."[27] It might have been the first such "experiment" anywhere in the world. Bright and the junior physician George H. Barlow took charge of the daily clinical conduct of the wards, including overseeing treatment, while three pupils wrote up cases in the traditional ward notebooks. George Owen Rees, Guy's physician and by then a thoroughly capable chemist, carried out the analyses of blood and urine. The team enjoyed the use of a room situated between the two wards "for the meeting of the Physicians and Pupils, and for the registry of the cases, and a small laboratory communicating with the middle room, fitted up and decorated entirely to our purpose." Bright stated that the "objects which we proposed to ourselves were, to examine, as far as possible, the changes which accompany the secretion of albuminous urine in the various functions and secretions of the body, whilst at the same time we registered the various circumstances connected with the origins, progress, and treatment of the disease."[28]

The cases from the summer experiment, described and tabulated with the chemical measurements made for some of the patients, filled over one hundred pages in the *Guy's Hospital Reports* of 1843. A few small and uncolored lithographic illustrations—clear and competently done but not at all dazzling—accompanied the text: attention had shifted from the pictorial to the numerical and chemical. But the overall effort still fell within the natural-historical manner of observing, noting, classifying, and reporting findings. The authors even took pains to affirm that they were "more anxious to furnish our readers with facts, than with any theories of our own."[29] The team did, however, organize some of the cases by the dominant therapy applied—mercurials, elaterium, antimonials, venesection, or "tonics." But the reader is left to judge the relative effectiveness of these measures (the cases were not all fatal).

So one might conclude that the organization of the summer study of renal disease at Guy's—the convening of a team, the dedication of beds, the ward laboratory—emerges as more remarkable than the additional knowledge accrued. How influential this experiment may have been in stimulating the idea of the metabolic research ward in hospitals is unknown. It is doubtful that any such arrangement took shape again until the late nineteenth century or beyond, and England was not destined to become the center of laboratory medicine. In fact, the chemical analysis of blood necessarily declined during the later nineteenth century with the reduced reliance on therapeutic bleeding to provide the samples. It did not revive until analytic methods were invented in the early decades of the twentieth century that could be used with small quantities of blood obtained by pinprick or a small syringe and needle. The kidneys are indeed chemical devices, responsible not only for excreting waste substances but also for the regulation of the bodily content of substances such as water, sodium, potassium, hydrogen ion (acid), and bicarbonate (alkali). Eventually, the measurement of these and other substances became inseparable from the study of renal function and renal disease.

In the mid-twentieth century and beyond, research physicians with interest in the kidney would again fashion themselves into chemists or ally themselves with those trained in the discipline. Of course, as medical science grew in theoretical and technical sophistication, collaboration of the physician and scientist became the necessary rule, as did organized investigation of disease in space set up for the purpose. We see at least a tantalizing foreshadowing of this at Guy's Hospital, during the first decades of Bright's Disease.

No doubt, many people with dropsy before the early 1800s had albuminuria and underlying kidney disease, but they did not have Bright's Disease. Bright's Disease could exist as a sickness entity and a diagnosis only within a particular context: it required the rise of large hospitals made subject, at least in part, to the curiosity and investigational intentions of physicians; a fervor for doing autopsies and in this way remapping diseases—and, frankly, a hospital mortality rate capable of providing the autopsies; possibly even an eagerness to depict nature as faithfully and colorfully as paints and paper would allow. Bright's Disease, therefore, awaited not so much Richard Bright—to whom credit is due—but to the convergence of these and perhaps other favorable circumstances. The experiment of assigning two wards and a laboratory to the study of renal disease at Guy's required other, some quite local, factors: the use of therapeutic letting of blood to make it available for analysis, an identifiable corps of "medical chemists," and a hospital–medical school eager to advance itself in a scientific direction following a reorganization. Certainly of fundamental importance at Guy's was a sort of spirit of investigation within an environment of collegiality.

Bright's way of doing clinical-pathological correlation was entirely of its day, while the prospective study with laboratory and chemical measurement hinted at the future. In that future, the sensory experiences and statements of patients would further yield authority to information produced by examination of the body, its blood, urine, and other fluids. But Bright and his colleagues confronted sick Londoners in their present. The doctors needed to make some sense of the "new" disease and select treatments. This required a foundation, a reliable structure well rooted in medicine's past. Such a need arises with the initial recognition or actual new appearance of a disease entity—therapy cannot await a novel theoretical formulation.[30] Bright's way of placing albuminuric renal disease into the knowledge structure and therapeutics of his time will make his medical world seem, to the twenty-first-century reader, primitive and strange. That is, if a medical reader of this book could be back in the 1830s, "rounding" at Guy's Hospital, the patients' stories, ward life, physical examinations, autopsies, and even laboratory would probably all seem at least recognizable, occasionally even familiar. But Bright's notions of causation, pathophysiological mechanism, and treatment would signal a distant and foreign land, which we shall enter in chapter 3.

―――∞∞――――

A Later Perspective

Proteinuria, the leakage of blood protein, mostly albumin, into the urine occurs mainly when some disease has altered the filtering properties of the glomerulus, the specialized tuft of capillaries and surrounding capsule described in chapter 1 and shown in the second figure in that chapter. These capillaries in sum can be thought of as a filtering membrane or sieve. Ordinarily, as blood flows through the glomeruli, they let pass into the fluid that will become urine almost all the dissolved substances in the blood plasma except the proteins. One reason is that most blood proteins are too large to pass through the exceedingly fine pores and "slits" in the membrane. These various proteins must be retained because they carry out a variety of necessary functions within the body. One such protein, and the one most subject to leakage from blood into the urine, is albumin. It can be detected in urine by heat coagulation (no longer used), by precipitation (coagulation) with acid (which Bright and contemporaries also employed), and now by a variety of quantitative techniques. Most often in current practice, it will first be discovered through use of the urine "dipstick," a plastic strip with a series of pads containing reagents that will turn color in the presence of glucose, protein, and so on.

When a renal disease has caused the glomeruli to be severely "leaky" to blood proteins, a complex of findings results known as the nephrotic syndrome. As noted at the end of chapter 1, somehow the reduction in the amount of blood albumin triggers a process by which the kidney retains salt and water far beyond bodily need, leading to edema and ascites, or dropsy in the old language. A lesser degree of albuminuria will not do this and was long thought of as merely a "marker" or indicator of renal disease, as indeed it is. Recent research, however, sees the movement of albumin across the overly porous glomerular membranes as itself harmful and responsible for further damage to the nephron units. Therefore, drugs known as angiotensin converting enzyme inhibitors, or ACE inhibitors, and angiotensin receptor blockers, or ARBs, have come into wide use for patients with some forms of chronic proteinuric kidney disease because they reduce the protein leakage and help prevent the further deterioration of kidney structure and function. They also lower elevated blood pressure and serve to protect impaired kidneys in other ways as well. The importance of these drugs in renal disease will be further described in chapter 9.

Paradoxically, even when a serious kidney disease has made the glomeruli overly permeable, or leaky, to proteins, such that albumin is easily detected in the urine, the overall loss of working nephron units can mean that the kidneys as a whole fail to adequately place into the urine what they normally should. Thus, with progressive renal disease of almost any type, substances excreted by the kidneys, such as urea, creatinine, potassium, and phosphate, will be retained in the body. Not all of these have been so far mentioned, but urea, as we have seen, was the first that could be detected in elevated amounts in the blood of renal patients by Bright's chemist friends. Now, measuring urea and creatinine in the blood is a critical part of detecting impairment of kidney function.

The retention of some toxic substances not adequately excreted by diseased kidneys leads to the syndrome of uremia (exactly which substances are most critical remains uncertain—probably urea and creatinine are not themselves very injurious). Furthermore, the kidneys play an important role in the regulation of blood pressure and in the control of the production of red blood cells. Bright did not use the term "uremia" but saw and described almost all its elements. Some "uremic toxin" presumably causes the inflammation (a word Bright did use) of certain "serous" or "lining" membranes of the body, and this can cause chest pain (pericarditis) and abdominal pain (peritonitis). "Inflammation" denotes that process in an organ or tissue of the body that reacts to some microbial infection, irritating stimulus, or injury and is marked typically by swelling, pain and tenderness, increased blood flow, and sometimes the appearance of pus. "Inflammation" is a term losing some of its utility in the age of molecular medicine but remains a familiar phenomenon to anyone who has had a sore throat, burn, "red eye," or tendonitis.

In uremia, some retained toxin also either irritates the stomach or influences certain centers in the brain stem, so that nausea and vomiting are frequent complaints in serious renal disease. Either retained toxins, or maybe retained water causing edema of the brain, or some combination of these, leads to the seizures described in some of the Guy's patients, another late event in renal disease. Seizures are now rarely seen because patients usually receive therapy with an artificial kidney before the onset of the most perilous symptoms. The "sharp" or "hard" pulse Bright and his colleagues could feel no doubt represented the elevated blood pressure that often accompanies disease of the kidneys (practical devices for measuring the pressure of the blood entered medical practice in the 1890s). Bright also described the thickening of the heart muscle, which has "hypertrophied" from overwork as it pumped against an elevated pressure. The shortness of breath that agonized some of Bright's patients was probably the same phenomenon seen in the earlier descriptions of dropsy: retained salt and water either pooling in the pleural space between the lung and inner chest wall (and thus placing pressure on the lungs), or excess water filling the lung itself.

Finally, the kidneys produce a hormonal substance called erythropoietin, which stimulates the bone marrow to produce red blood cells at a rate adjusted to keep their number in the blood within a normal range; red cells, of course, deliver oxygen to tissues and cells. Any form of chronic kidney disease can, in its advanced stage, lead to insufficient production of erythropoietin. The body becomes deficient in circulating red cells (anemic), with consequent fatigue, headache, and pallor. Bright saw the pallor, and his laboratory friends showed the decreased amount of red cells in the blood. Beginning in the 1980s, a synthetic form of erythropoietin became available as an injectable medication. Although expensive, it has proved of great value in correcting the anemia of persons with advanced chronic renal disease, restoring to them at least some of their previous vigor.

CHAPTER THREE

Sympathy and Flannel

—◦◦◦—

Richard Bright worked in what one might with some understatement term a vigorously therapeutic medical world, at a hospital that held the reputation for particular forcefulness in the treatment of disease. It was not a time, or a place, that much championed the healing power of nature. Furthermore, Bright's first renal patients at Guy's Hospital exuded florid sickness, the sort that seemed to demand that something be done. Bright found a way to understand his new disease and treat it using what was available to him—a time-honored, even ancient, set of explanatory concepts that seemed to fit the circumstances preceding the individual's illnesses. In addition, the title he gave his great book promised a "view of illustrating the symptoms *and cure* of diseases by a reference to morbid anatomy" (emphasis mine)—morbid anatomy, the pathological alterations found at the *sectio cadaveris,* might offer therapeutic guidance, not just theoretical ideas about where sickness is situated in the body. Paradoxically, of course, no one who could contribute such therapeutic insights had been cured, but Bright believed the process could lead to progress.

Here are some of Dr. Bright's words, which told his readers where he thought albuminuric renal disease came from, what its "mechanism" was, and how one should treat it:

An intemperate course of life, or some such cause, has predisposed the kidney to suffer. The patient has, in this state, been exposed to vicissitudes of temperature; the irritable kidney has immediately sympathized with the skin, and morbid action has been induced in that organ; the balance of absorption has been destroyed, and serous accumulations have taken place. . . . If the kidneys have previously been healthy, and if the patient be seen early, and antiphlogistic remedies actively employed, the morbid action subsides; the urine ceases to be coagulable, the anasarca disappears, and the patient is perfectly restored, without any organic lesion of the kidney. (Written in 1833)[1]

In the treatment of this formidable disease, in the early periods of its attack, I look to the circumstances with which it is most frequently connected—I mean the suppression of the perspiration, and the consequent general inflammatory condition—as most important. (1836)[2]

Sympathy. Suppressed perspiration. What is Bright talking about here?[3] Since at least the time of the Graeco-Roman physician Galen, it was held that suppression of the "insensible perspiration"—the movement of water vapor across skin—could have dangerous consequences. Certain organs displayed "sympathy" with each other, a kind of special connection or interdependence, such that an injury or irritation of one would lead to dysfunction of the other. The skin sympathized with the stomach, and both might with the kidney. "Checking" the exhalatory function of the skin by chilling it—suppressing the insensible perspiration—could therefore lead to congestion and even inflammation in the kidney. ("Congestion" refers to a local area of excess blood flow and accumulation of blood, the "redness" component of inflammation.) In a woman, sudden cessation or "suppression" of the menses could also cast remote effects through sympathy. Bright, or any physician of his time, inherited these versatile old concepts, and not as hypotheses or speculation, but as unshakable *knowledge* of how things worked in disease. Furthermore, he repeatedly saw this process play out in those under care at Guy's.

From the *Reports of Medical Cases:* bricklayer Daniel Peacock (case 4) had become hot from "carrying a great weight . . . drank some cold beer and lay on the damp grass;—the following day, or the day after, his legs began to swell." Henry Izod (case 11), the "Smithfield drover," was "accustomed to get intoxicated with porter . . . and had been much exposed in his work to the inclemency of the weather; seldom wearing a hat, never changing his clothes when wet." Leonard Evans (case 14), the "strongest man out of 1400 in Deptford dockyard . . . has often been exposed to cold, when in a state of most profuse perspiration." His swelling came on the same day his feet became exceptionally wet.[4] From Bright's 1836 article in *Guy's Hospital Reports,* we hear of case 5, "Mr. P, an athletic young man of 25 years of age, by trade a plumber," who, when already feeling ill with dyspepsia, still went on top of a building to supervise some work, where he was "exposed to the weather; and returned home ill, as if from cold."[5] And one could go on. No doubt many of Bright's working-class patients at Guy's did drink, and none worked at a desk comfortably warmed by a fireplace. Bright, or his pupils, heard the sufferer's history ("took the case") and over and over again could uncover a story of inebriety, wetness, and cold among those with "renal dropsy."

We might pause here to suggest that the identification of these episodes of soak and chill, beyond confirming medical theory and informing treatment, served another essential need within the old enterprise of ill person, doctor, and disease. The stories allowed physician and the sick man or woman *to make sense of what had happened:* to place the onset of illness within the context of the life daily lived, within a framework of order, and even within a moral universe. Clinicians know that persons newly ill want to know "why did this happen to *me?*" even to the extent of trying to recall some blameworthy misstep or failing that might have led to getting sick. And physicians also have taken comfort in some logical tale of cause and effect, though sometimes too readily assigning fault to the patient.

This desire to identify a causal story may have been especially entrenched before the relatively recent willingness to think in statistical terms and accept the idea of randomness—that even among persons "predisposed," only some few in a given year will be struck with pneumonia, or gout, or cancer. Even the ancient case narratives from the Hippocratic writings show this. We can read (in *Epidemics III*) that the "lad who lay by the Liars' Market took a fever as the result of exhaustion, having exerted himself by running more than he was accustomed," or that "the wife of Delearces, who lay on the level ground, took a high fever with shivering as the result of grief." And, of course, there would be "a young man who had been running a temperature for a long time as the result of drinking and much sexual indulgence."[6]

Bright's stories of albuminous dropsy show that some of those under his care were exposed to chill in their hard work and could not avoid it. Others brought misfortune on themselves through carelessness, or—worse—inebriety. In either case, an expectation of rationality or even moral balance is fulfilled. In London of the 1820s, one did not get deadly sick by chance, or through the whim of a deity.[7] Persons with Bright's Disease never would, however, suffer the stigma of contagion, since it was never deemed transmissible from one person to another. And, by the twentieth century, it even lost its association with inebriety.

Among Bright's patients, that suppression of the skin's activity by a chill (however acquired) had induced internal irritation or inflammation in various organs found confirmation not only in the abnormal secretion by the kidneys of albumin and occasionally red blood cells but also in the inflammatory symptoms, such as pleuritic chest pains, abdominal pains, and even convulsions. Also, autopsy could show the actual pathological indicators of inflammation as seen in the pericardium, pleura, and sometimes the kidneys.[8] To reduce the inflammation and congestion, consequences of an excess level of "action" to which the body seemed pitched by the disease, Bright in acute cases relied on what were considered "antiphlogistic" (anti-inflammatory) and "depleting" measures. Among these were bloodletting, though Bright tended to bleed less as he gained years of experience with renal disease. He did use purgatives freely, and—in keeping with traditional ways of lessening dropsy—sometimes drugs that were considered diuretics and diaphoretics.

We may recall from chapter 2 Thomas Drudget, the carman and good family man, case 13 from the *Reports of Medical Cases*.[9] His renal disease presented first with nausea, vomiting, and shortness of breath, then with dropsy in the legs. Bright reported no exposure to cold or wet. Still, to the physician the symptoms and the coagulable urine pointed to a pattern, part of which was inflammation. To reduce the inflammatory component, Bright ordered repeated bloodletting using the technique of "cupping," applied to the patient's skin over the chest and over the low back, corresponding to the region of the kidneys.[10] He also used calomel (a mercurial drug, considered an antiphlogistic and also a cathartic and diuretic), then preparations containing magnesium sulphate, camphor, and potassium supertartrate, as cathartics and diuretics. Bright repeated cupping over the kidneys and later in the hospital course ordered jalap (another cathartic-diuretic, long favored for dropsy). He made his daily therapeutic decisions based on the patients' responses and what he found on examination, though the modern reader cannot follow the logic—why add jalap now? Why no further calomel?

On the evening of the eleventh day of hospitalization, Drudget complained of headache. "About eight o'clock it was observed that he lay in bed making a very singular noise, and on going to him he was in a state of profound apoplectic stertor. Mr. Stocker was immediately called; took away twenty ounces of blood from the temporal artery, gave him ten grains of calomel, and a colocynth injection. He had one or two fresh attacks, accompanied with so much convulsion that he could scarcely be held in bed."[11] (Stocker was the Guy's apothecary, a practitioner serving as a kind of on-call house doctor.) Bright ordered more bloodletting, a dose of croton oil (a ferocious cathartic), an enema, and a cantharides plaster (Spanish fly, a "counterirritant") to the neck, but to no avail: Drudget died . . . and contributed his kidneys to the emerging knowledge of renal pathology. Many of the drugs and even the cupping used in his management had been employed for dropsy before it had been linked to disturbed kidneys. Bright and his colleagues could not, of course, treat the very sick in a therapeutic vacuum—they could not formulate entirely novel remedies because they were dealing with a new disease. But at least some of the choices—cupping over the kidneys and the vigorous antiphlogistic measures—derived from the knowledge that *this* case of dropsy was connected with disease in the *kidney,* and from a conceptualization of the underlying pathological process (inflammation or congestion).

BRIGHT'S CARE FOR THE CHRONIC CASE

Once Bright had gained experience with more mild and chronic cases, which probably have always outnumbered the very acute forms, he could make recommendations for them. Convinced that a chill, through suppressing the "perspirability" of the skin, set into motion the pathophysiological events causing albuminous renal disease, he declared the importance of keeping the subject warm: "On the subject of clothing I have already said all that is necessary: let flannel be worn constantly, and every precaution be habitually adopted which may obviate the effects of whatever is calculated to chill the surface or check the perspiration."[12]

And although recognizing that "the disease being, unfortunately, most apt to occur in those least able to submit to the absence from business," he advised in his 1836 article that removal to "some decidedly southern abode. . . . One of the more healthy of the West-India islands, as St. Vincent's, would probably be beneficial."[13] Bright admitted that he so far had not encountered any patient who could actually manage this recommendation, which of course long had been applied to dropsy; we saw that Henry Fielding's ascites sent him to Lisbon. Nineteenth-century physicians urged travel for other chronic diseases, particularly consumption, something like the antithesis of dropsy. Consumptives of means would travel to wherever was sunnier, usually south, or take bracing sea voyages, whereas the poor might be dispatched to a sanatorium on the nearest mountainside, far enough from their city neighborhood to feel lonely. Those tormented with hay fever or asthma journeyed in season to find relieving mountain airs.[14] Well before this, throughout the later Middle Ages, the lame, blind, deaf, and other long-sufferers of Europe sought cure through pilgrimage to the shrine of a healing saint, usually the one voyage of their wretched lives.

We can follow the first authority's management of a more indolent case of Bright's Disease by examining case 4 of his "Memoir the Second" of 1840.[15] The subject of the report, presumably from Bright's private practice, and for whom no name is listed, was a "man, aged about 25, pale and scrofulous in appearance, and deeply pitted with the small-pox," who, in early March of 1835, "came to me, labouring under anasarca, and having albuminous urine." His illness began with diarrhea eight months before that lasted three weeks. As he recovered, the young man was able to spend a month in the country, but there "his legs began to swell, and anasarca proceeded up his thighs and abdomen." Bright found the urine "exceedingly coagulable" and "frothy on agitation" (frothy or sudsy urine can indicate the presence of albumin). The man tended to pass large, not small, quantities of urine. "I ordered him to adopt most strictly a milk diet, and to put on warm clothing, with flannel next to the skin." Because the stomach "sympathized" with the skin and kidneys, its irritability had to be quieted with an easy diet and gentle medicines such as bicarbonate of soda, which Bright prescribed. He also gave humulus and uva ursi, both plant-derived medicines with supposed general "tonic" and perhaps diuretic properties. Some ipecac was also called for as a mild emetic or diaphoretic.

The man improved briefly, with less coagulability of the urine, but in April developed some cough, and his "skin inclined to be dry." Bright prescribed again some ipecac, which in smaller dose was used as a diaphoretic and expectorant. By June the gentleman had improved greatly, his swelling almost gone, though the urine still "froths much." Then a painful "periosteal enlargement" appeared on his left shin, which the patient feared was the reappearance of "some venereal symptoms," presumably syphilis. Bright prescribed a concoction for this. By July 9 the man was again "greatly improved" and the reader now learns that he was a bookbinder and was able to return to work. This seemed to signify for the physician (and presumably the patient) an objective and decisive indicator of improved health. He now slept well and was not dropsical, but the urine still frothed and coagulated when tested. Bright desired him "to persist in all his cares and precautions [the restricted diet and flannel on the skin], to abstain from all spirits, and carefully avoid atmospheric exposures." He continued the mixture of ipecac, bicarbonate of soda, and uva ursi as the primary medication, presumably aimed at keeping the urine flowing, the skin moist, the stomach calm, and at fulfilling the imperative that medicine be prescribed by the doctor, and that medicine be ingested by the patient.

In February of 1836, Bright "saw him casually," and found that he still worked and had "no complaint to make." But on questioning, the physician learned that the bookbinder now and then admitted to a slight headache. In addition, though neither his face nor ankles became puffy, the patient himself (who was a craftsman, worked with his hands) tested his ankles from time to time and found that sometimes they pitted to pressure of the finger. He slept well early in the night but became "restless" later and had to get up once to pass urine. The urine was "natural in quantity" and presumably looked normal, but both heat and nitric acid detected that it was still "very decidedly coagulable." Thus in the new sense (laboratory findings), disease persisted, though the man felt generally well. Importantly, the skin was "freely perspirable" and had been for so long "that he forgets it ever was otherwise." The young man had also ceased taking his medications regularly. The pox-marked bookbinder was choosing to further redefine himself as among the working nonsick. But if he felt some flank pain or noted some other hint of his complaints returning, he took the powders that Bright had prescribed for a few weeks, with "he fancies . . . the best effect." And he was always very careful to "guard his body with flannel next to the skin."

It is October 1839, and the gentleman consulted Bright after a four-year absence. He had continued in good health until three or four months before: he passed his time in the "comfortable discharge of his business," had no swelling, his skin function was "natural," and his urine of seemingly normal quantity. Lately, however, he suffered "frequent calls to pass it after going to bed"; and he complained of headache, nausea, and vomiting. A few days later Bright was able to test the urine: it coagulated slightly to heat, but readily with nitric acid. The bookbinder passed now "a large quantity of urine at night, but little in the day: his ankles had swollen slightly of late." Bright commented that "it is difficult to say" to what extent the medicines, or the precautionary measures of diet and clothing, contributed "to the relief of his disease." There is even a hint in Bright's words that the prescriber himself felt some skepticism about the power of the ipecac, bi-carbonate, and uva ursi. He pointed out that perhaps the decisive factor was that the skin remained "natural in its function," for although "a free perspiration by no means changes the nature of the urine, it appears to counteract in some degree the evils under which the constitution would otherwise be oppressed." And with this homage to the skin and endorsement of ancient medical doctrine, Bright concluded his patient's story, one that in many of its essentials faithfully represents chronic and slowly progressive proteinuric renal disease at any time.

In the study of the history of diseases and patients, we are usually limited, as with this case, to narratives created by the doctors. Samuel Johnson and Henry Fielding proved eloquent exceptions for an earlier period, and we shall see later that many persons with renal disease in the twentieth century living in dependence on the dialysis machine, or recipients of a kidney transplantation, felt impelled to write about their experiences. Bright's detailed case history at least conveys some sense of a young person living in a fairly tolerable degree of truce with his chronic disease—able to go about his life's work (we hear nothing of wife or family) and permit himself stretches in which he lay aside his medicines, the unmistakable and unpleasant markers of being sick. He also passed four years without seeing his "specialist" (we don't know if he consulted other doctors). But to wear flannel, occasionally pinch his ankles (hoping no pit will be seen), he can accept with equanimity.

It is doubtful that by the mid-1830s the diagnosis of Bright's Disease conveyed the gravity it would later, or conveyed much meaning at all to the diagnosed. We don't even know if this young man knew he had "Bright's Disease" in those words, or—if he did—what it felt like to have it managed by Bright! We also do not know with certainty the outcome, though the modern clinician can readily recognize that the most recent recurrence of headaches (elevated blood pressure?), vomiting, and edema portend the onset of terminal uremia. Or, perhaps not, in this only partly predictable disorder: he might enjoy yet another remission, if the skin and good fortune consent. We also see in this case narrative, and one might say appealingly for the most part, that Bright again situated the medical events within the complexities of a life lived, particularly the man's work. Also perceptible is the moral consideration always present to the Victorian physician—his patient's omitted medicines and failure to follow up, the specter of that "venereal complaint."

OTHER EARLY APPROACHES TO TREATMENT

The treatment of Bright's Disease remained remarkably unchanged for the next fifty years or more. James Tyson (1841–1919), an American authority on Bright's Disease, presented several cases to students on October 20, 1892, at University of Pennsylvania Hospital. One was a fifty-five-year-old woman whose massive "collection of fluid ruptured the skin. Today the leg is swollen, but is reduced though it still pits on pressure." She had albuminuria and granular casts (formed elements indicative of renal disease) in the urine, and was treated with a milk diet and with caffeine as a diuretic. Tyson sometimes used pilocarpine to induce a sweat, and often a device he seemed to cherish called the "hot-air bath," a contrivance for delivering warmed air to a patient wrapped in blankets—all aimed at activating the skin. On October 27, 1892, Tyson discussed a young man with acute Bright's Disease, who on "the way home from the West took cold and developed severe bronchitis." Tyson, like Bright fifty years earlier, still saw cold as a common cause of albuminuric renal disease, and treated accordingly. In his book on Bright's Disease of 1881 he recommended "residence in a warm equable climate" and recounted how one "lady past middle age" with granular kidneys felt "like a young girl" during a stay in a warm area of southern Germany only to promptly regain her symptoms upon landing in chilly Liverpool on her way home to the United States. Tyson also resorted to venesection in refractory cases.[16]

William Osler, a leading internist, teacher, and medical scholar of the late nineteenth and early twentieth centuries, in the 1905 edition of his widely used *Principles and Practice of Medicine* devoted much detail to the treatment of chronic Bright's Disease. Osler, even more than Bright, reflected back to a Hippocratic idea of "regimen," the complete management of diet and life activities. He recommended "a quiet life without mental worry, with gentle

but not excessive exercise, and residence in an equable climate"
(he presumably had read Tyson's work), such as Southern California. The bowels should be kept regular and the "skin active."
The diet must be "light and nourishing" and for acute cases he
recommended milk, as did other authorities. For the dropsy and
increased arterial tension (by then, blood pressure measurement
was possible), Osler in 1905 called for sweating the patient with
hot baths or hot air. For uremic convulsions, chloroform can be
tried (unknown to Bright), but from a "robust and full-blooded"
person, "12 to 20 ounces of blood should be removed."[17]

By 1905, the microscope had revised the categorization of
Bright's Disease, and several specific causes had been identified.
But, as generally has been the case in the history of therapeutics,
treatment lagged behind advance in theory. Time-proven measures seem to work, and sometimes new theories of mechanism
or causation fall into place in ways to explain the efficacy of the
seasoned and familiar remedies. Chapter 4 will drop back to look
more fully at the changes in the understanding of Bright's Disease
that occurred during the hundred years following Bright's discoveries.

A Later Perspective

The conviction that excess drinking of alcohol could lead to kidney
disease persisted into the early twentieth century; oddly enough,
the kidney is now believed to be one of the few organs not subject
to the widespread ill effects of inebriety. Of course, the pervasive
belief that "suppression of the insensible perspiration" could cause
internal disease now resides within the history of medicine, a fine
exemplar of the fickleness of truth. Cold as a cause of kidney disease persisted as a medical, then popular, concept at least into
the 1920s: a senior physician told me that Philadelphia children
were once warned against sitting outside on a chilly night with
their backs against the cold stone row-house steps because doing
so might bring on nephritis. In general, the timeless connection
between cold or a chill and getting sick probably has its basis in
infectious disease. A chill precedes a fever and can in fact be considered part of the mechanism that generates the fever. A chill can

certainly mark the onset of a streptococcal sore throat or streptococcal scarlet fever, and certain members of this species of bacteria
can induce an immunological reaction causing "postinfectious" or
"poststreptococcal" glomerulonephritis. (The ending "-itis" continues to denote an inflammatory condition, with glomerulonephritis
an inflammation of the glomerular ball of capillaries.) No doubt
some cases of "acute Bright's Disease" represented poststreptococcal glomerulonephritis, as did the "dropsy which follows scarlatina,"
which Bright and his predecessors encountered and wrote about.
This disease continues to occur sporadically or in occasional outbreaks.

The nineteenth-century treatment of inflammatory (or "phlo-
gistic") disorders with bloodletting, mercury preparations, laxatives, and emetics has been replaced, thankfully, by agents such
as aspirin, nonsteroidal anti-inflammatory drugs (NSAIDs), cortisone, and newer "designer" medications that interfere with some
of the molecular or cellular mediators of inflammation. Inflammation brought on by disturbances in the body's immunologic systems underlies many forms of glomerulonephritis and other proteinuric kidney disease as now understood, and drugs related to
cortisone, as well as others that reduce the action of overactive
immune processes, are frequently called upon. For example, prednisone is a drug in the class called glucocorticoids, which includes
cortisone, first brought into clinical use in the late 1940s for rheu-
matoid arthritis. Prednisone is used to treat the glomerulonephritis
that sometimes forms a part of the disease systemic lupus erythematosus, or "lupus," a disorder of immune regulation that particularly afflicts young women. In current medical practice, statistically
analyzed "clinical trials" support the worth of such treatments in
a manner unknown, or only hinted at, before about 1950. So we
feel confident that they work—though possibly, no more confident
than Bright, Tyson, or Osler felt about their therapeutic options.
And the drugs currently used exhibit toxicities, as did their now
derided predecessors.

Sweating, whether brought on by a drug, a "hot-air bath," flannel, or a stay in a region of warm climate, can—as already discussed—help reduce the dropsy, or edema, associated with some
renal diseases, because it will reduce the body's excess burden of salt

and water. But this strategy is rarely resorted to now. Some of the drugs the nineteenth-century physicians used as diuretics (agents that stimulate the kidneys to excrete salt and water) may indeed have had such an effect, though there is no way to be certain, since no one particularly wishes to revive them and study their effects. Bright for his chronic patient made sodium bicarbonate part of his three-drug "powders," aiming the bicarbonate at relieving stomach symptoms. It may have done this, and, unbeknownst to Bright, the bicarbonate, an alkaline salt, would have helped combat the excess acidification of the blood that almost invariably occurs in advanced chronic renal disease (referred to as "metabolic acidosis"). The body produces acid as it utilizes ingested protein, especially protein derived from meat, and the kidneys serve the function of excreting the acid in the urine as they produce fresh bicarbonate to "buffer" the acid in the body. Renal patients of the twenty-first century may still include sodium bicarbonate in their long lists of medications, though a closely related liquid alkaline preparation of sodium citrate is now preferred. Untreated, metabolic acidosis can lead to loss of calcium from bones, and—when severe enough—a distressing sensation of hunger for air.

CHAPTER FOUR

Enter the Microscope
and the Laboratory

———◦◦◦———

With the work of Bright and his British colleagues, then Europeans such as the Frenchman Pierre Rayer,[1] the kidney now occupied a secure location within the table of contents of diseases. But even Bright could not be sure that Bright's Disease was in fact one entity. His numerous postmortem observations led him to see three distinct pathological variants: a soft, yellow-mottled kidney of normal size; a kidney showing a "granulated texture" and also some sort of whitish deposit; and a form in which the kidney is "rough and scabrous to the touch," "lobulated," and shows numerous "yellow, red, and purplish" pinhead-size projections over the surface.[2] The first illustration discussed in chapter 2 represents the second form. Future nephrologists (the name assumed since the 1960s by physicians specializing in renal disease) looking back at Bright's *Reports of Medical Cases* would find themselves perplexed that Bright displayed, but did not explicitly categorize, other forms—a large, swollen red kidney, engorged with blood (the second figure in chapter 2) and a large, pale white kidney. He could not be sure if there were three different diseases leading to albuminuria and dropsy or whether he was merely coming upon one disease at various stages.

Pathology, and especially the classification of diseases and "lesions" (a general term for pathological alterations in organs or tissues), continued as the source of much medical investigation of the nineteenth century. Three advances moved the center of pathology from the appearance of the whole organ, which Bright examined, to the microscopic level: improvements in the optics and ease of use of the microscope (1830s), the emergence of the cell theory (1830s–1850s), and the application of staining methods for microscopy, to better distinguish among types of cells (1850s and 1860s).[3] By the 1840s, the refined microscope was focused on kidneys with Bright's Disease, still obtained at autopsy, and begat a series of classifications.[4] For many decades, controversy continued about the "unity" of Bright's Disease: was there indeed but one disease, each case moving in time through a fixed clinical and pathological natural history? Or did Bright's Disease comprise multiple disease entities—the viewpoint that eventually prevailed? Friedrich Theodor von Frerichs (1819–1885) of the Charité Hospital in Berlin, a prominent figure in German internal medicine and pathology, analyzing his own cases and those published before him, proposed three microscopically separable stages of one disease.[5] But most physician-pathologists favored the belief that Bright's Disease really comprised many variants.

The story of the superceding and competing classifications is far too complex and tedious to narrate except in the broadest of strokes. Oddly, nephrologists and pathologists looking at altered kidneys have always favored as much as possible a tripartite organization, either seeking simplicity or emulating Dr. Bright. Rudolph Virchow (1821–1902), the giant of German medicine and public health who pushed the study of disease to the level of the cell, in 1858 suggested: "parenchymatous nephritis," "interstitial nephritis," and "amyloid degeneration."[6] George Johnson (1818–1896), physician to King's College Hospital in London, and a major British contributor to renal medicine after Bright, in 1873 proposed the separation of an acute form ("acute nephritis") and three chronic varieties: "red granular kidney," "large white kidney," and "lardaceous kidney" (which is the same as the "amyloid" variant).[7] William Osler in his influential *Principles and Practice of Medicine*, first published in 1892, favored "acute Bright's disease," "chronic parenchymatous nephritis," and "chronic interstitial nephritis," with "amyloid" dispatched to its own pathological category.

Into the twentieth century, the extremely influential monograph by Germans Franz Volhard (1872–1950) and Theodor Fahr (1877–1945) published in 1914, *Die Brightsche Nierenkrankheit* (*Bright's Disease of the Kidney*), provided a fresh—but still trinitarian—organization: inflammatory diseases, the "nephritides"; degenerative diseases, the "nephroses"; and arteriosclerotic diseases, the "nephroscleroses."[8] Scotsman Thomas Addis (1881–1949), an expert in kidney disease who spent most of his career at Stanford University, in the 1920s offered a modification of this last framework that gained some popularity: "hemorrhagic Bright's disease," "degenerative Bright's disease," and "arteriosclerotic Bright's disease." Volhard and Fahr in Germany and Addis in California derived their claims for the "real" categories of Bright's Disease from classical clinical-pathological correlation using autopsies (but applying the microscope); these were among the last major figures to work in that tradition.[9]

What sense can be made of these arcane names and classifications? All the classifiers seemed to agree that there was an acute form that made urine bloody as well as albuminuric, caused pain in the kidney area (the flanks), and was associated with a blood-engorged, swollen kidney. This later became known as acute glomerulonephritis (or glomerular nephritis) and represents an inflammatory process attacking the glomeruli, sometimes following a streptococcal infection; it was the "dropsy which follows scarlatina" that Richard Bright and his predecessors had recognized, though about which Bright said little, even though he showed an example in his colored plates. Various names were assigned to a form of Bright's Disease marked dominantly by *extreme* albuminuria, associated mainly with stubborn dropsy, or edema: the kidney is often large and pale. This later became known as nephrotic syndrome. The microscope and a growing awareness of chronic disease of blood vessels, eventually to be linked to high blood pressure and cholesterol, led to the category of arteriosclerotic diseases—Bright's Disease arising from narrowing and "hardening" of the kidney's arterial network. The microscope also identified a pattern of a seemingly starchlike, or amyloid, deposition in the glomeruli, distinctive enough to form a separate category. It came to be associated with long-standing, smoldering inflammatory disease elsewhere in the body—for example, tuberculosis or certain types of arthritis.

By the 1920s, physicians and pathologists studying renal diseases had moved much of their attention to the glomerulus, the globular filtering apparatus at the head of each nephron unit. It comprises the tuft of blood-filtering capillaries, and the "cup" of the tubule into which the glomerular products—the filtered fluid and accompanying dissolved substances—flow (see the second figure in chapter 1). This shift in focus followed the lead of the very influential Franz Volhard, already mentioned, the leading German authority on renal disease of the early twentieth century. Microscopic analyses by Volhard and others came up with varieties of glomerulonephritis beyond the poststreptococcal type mentioned previously. These won such names as "focal," "embolic-focal," and "diffuse" (including "subacute diffuse" and "chronic diffuse"). In fact, by the 1920s "glomerulonephritis" began to displace the well-aged but not very scientific-sounding "Bright's Disease" (though not all that had been called Bright's Disease was glomerulonephritis).[10]

Thus, later nineteenth-century and early twentieth-century physicians and pathologists interested in Bright's Disease relied primarily on microscopic pathology to "spin out" an increasingly detailed categorization, or nosography, of the disorder. Looking back, one can pick out the concepts that would endure (such as amyloidosis of the kidneys, glomerulonephritis, and vascular disease), some that would serve as forerunners of "our current understanding," and other categories that no longer exist. But that is not the main point. A physician and historian named Knud Faber has said about disease categories that the clinician "cannot live, cannot speak, cannot act without them."[11] They organize thinking and teaching about diseases, and a classification system in itself becomes one form of mastery over what previously had been confused or mysterious. In this latter sense, the classification of diseases can be seen as part of the process of "taming" nature, in the same way that botanists created orderly arrangements for the kingdom of plants. In fact, the classification of diseases and of plants and animals went on at the same time, in part by the same persons, since many physicians in Great Britain and Europe were also skilled naturalists.

For ill persons and doctors, of course, classification held practical value. It placed the sick person in a framework of medical understandings and actions, as Faber implied. As with earlier systems of medical thought, the classification of Bright's Disease, once something like a reasonable consensus existed, succeeded in answering questions physicians needed to ask. Both prognosis and treatment might depend upon correctly determining the variant of a disease afflicting a particular individual—if it could be determined other than by postmortem examination.

Furthermore, labor at the microscope constituted a desirable form of professional work within medical science by the second half of the nineteenth century, particularly in Germany. There, in contrast to the England of Richard Bright in the 1830s and 1840s, a career in medical research could exist within the universities. Although "Bright's Disease" still held meaning and utility as a disease entity in itself, the physician-pathologists breaking it down into smaller pathological units were inching toward a more esoteric, even specialist, understanding. As we will see in chapter 5, this movement accelerated with the advent of the renal biopsy— the ability to apply microscopic analysis to renal tissue obtained from the living patient—as well as other sorts of refined investigation in the laboratory.

NOT ALWAYS FROM A CHILL

Even well into the twentieth century, "cold" continued to serve as a cause of Bright's Disease, at least the acute form, and it was widely believed that the acute form could evolve into the chronic variety. With the coming of the germ theory in the 1860s and beyond, what had been known as the "dropsy which follows scarlatina," then acute hemorrhagic Bright's Disease, was understood as a consequence of infection of the throat or skin by the streptococcal bacteria (later poststreptococcal glomerulonephritis). Similarly, infections such as malaria and syphilis were recognized to occasionally trigger acute Bright's Disease. The cause of the chronic, and often insidious, cases of albuminuric renal disease often remained a mystery when a patient had suffered no evident attack of the acute form. Sometimes, chronic cases were deemed a complication of gout. Gout in earlier times showed many faces, refused confinement to the big toe, and accepted blame for all manner of complaints.[12] But it was in good part the inability to identify a preceding cause for most cases of chronic Bright's Disease that required the classification schemes to rest mainly on the visual appearance, with the attendant risk of subjectivity, or errors of either too much "lumping" or "splitting."

By the 1880s, for the first time, an occupational exposure achieved a fixed place in the widening categorization of Bright's Disease, namely, "plumbism," or lead poisoning. James Tyson, the expert on Bright's Disease from Philadelphia encountered earlier, believed that the lead in the blood "excites the proliferating activity of the connective tissue elements [of the kidney]. Hence, painters, glaziers, workers in lead in any shape, are frequent victims."[13] Later, lead-induced renal disease was identified among children in Queensland, Australia, who chewed flaking lead paint on the verandahs of their homes, and in habitual imbibers of homemade "moonshine" in the American south. The clandestine distillation apparatus often contributed lead from solder joints to the drink; some adherents asserted that the lead salt that formed actually leant the beverage a certain sweetness. Here again Bright's Disease, as with any ailment, revealed its situation within particular social or cultural circumstances. By 1905, William Osler and others explored another form of environmental, even "psychosocial," cause of renal disease. Osler wrote that the "arterio-sclerotic form" was the most common type in the United States, seen in "men over forty who have worked hard, eaten freely, and taken alcohol to excess." They are "conspicuous victims of the 'strenuous life,' the incessant tension of which is felt first in the arteries. After forty in men of this class nothing is more salutary than to experience the shock brought by the knowledge of the presence of albumin and tube-casts in the urine. The associated cardio-vascular changes are of varying degrees of intensity, and upon them, not upon the renal condition, does the outlook depend."[14]

Here, in discussing Bright's Disease, Osler offered a concise premonition of one of the notable medical-moral tales of the industrial age, at least in the United States. In his abundant private practice, the revered doctor and teacher had cared for railroad presidents and captains of manufacture, who worked too hard, ate too richly, drank too much, and eventually confronted high blood pressure and its consequences in the kidney. The diagnosis of sickness in the kidneys, announced by signs in the urine, and no doubt at some point by the proclamation "Bright's Disease," can "shock" in a "salutary" manner. The hard-driving businessman need not have symptoms to hear the worrisome news: merely the protein in the urine and the "tube-casts" suffice to apply the label. But because symptoms may be few, there is still time to deal with the disordered renal organization. Doing so demands a moral and medical turnaround—medical in the old (Hippocratic) sense of "regimen," the health-building adjustment of diet, drink, sleep, and all activities. This albuminuric precursor of the later "Type A," wrote Osler, must reduce alcohol intake, tame gluttony, and tangle less in the brutal arena of American business of the industrial age.

TUBE-CASTS

What about those "tube-casts," whose presence along with some albumin in the urine might shock the captain of business into a more restrained mode of living? Urinary casts are microscopic cylinders of tissue debris and protein that result from inflammatory and degenerative renal diseases. They form within the renal tubules and wash out into the urine, where they become conveniently available for viewing under the microscope. Golding Bird (1815–1854), another Guy's physician, published a manual called *Urinary Deposits: Their Diagnosis, Pathology, and Therapeutical Indications* in 1844. It enjoyed numerous reprintings and editions, even after Bird's death. Similar manuals appeared in France and Germany also beginning in the 1840s. James Tyson of Philadelphia issued his *Guide to the Practical Examination of Urine* in 1875, and it found wide use (including a French translation) for over twenty-five years.[15] All later nineteenth-century manuals of this sort as well as texts on Bright's Disease contain extensive discussion of casts, often carefully illustrated by wood engravings. As with the classification of Bright's Disease itself, tube-casts became sorted into species—red cell casts, white cell casts, hyaline casts, granular casts, and so on. Connoisseurs of casts in the urine sought to link these various minute objects with the several categories of Bright's Disease. Thus, examination of the urinary sediment extended histological (microscopic) diagnosis to the living patient.[16] The ability to identify and interpret urinary casts and other findings entered the growing and increasingly specialized knowledge base surrounding Bright's Disease. Along with albuminuria, seeing casts in the urine also provided a circumstance in which physicians could declare a particular diagnosis for a patient who might lack symptoms pointing to the kidneys or who might lack any symptoms at all. Even more persuasively than albuminuria, the presence in the urine of granular casts came to signify the presence of some sort of mischief in the kidneys, a rule still in force as I write this in 2006.

FUNCTIONAL DIAGNOSIS AND BRIGHT'S DISEASE

Although pathology—altered structure—remained the underpinning of organized knowledge and diagnosis of Bright's Disease in the century after Bright, clinicians at the bedside of course continued to confront the symptoms and changes it caused in the functions of the human body—dropsy or edema (fluid retention), and uremia (the effects of retained toxins on the workings of brain, stomach, etc.). In the last decade of the nineteenth century and the early part of the twentieth, some investigators in Europe subjected Bright's Disease to a different sort of "functional diagnosis," using the laboratory. Functional diagnosis entailed the attempt to determine a diseased organ's capacity to carry out its biological tasks, or functions, rather than just to describe its altered appearance. Advocates of this approach, which arose in the 1870s mainly in the laboratories of Germany, devised ways to challenge or "stress" an organ, to see what it could or could not do.[17] How well could a sick stomach propel downstream a quantified "test meal" in comparison to a healthy one? How much might the ailing heart increase its pumping capacity when a subject exercised? Methods and thinking analogous to those applied to the stomach and heart were applied to the kidney.

In the late 1890s the Hungarian physician Sandor (or Alexander) von Koranyi (1866–1944) measured the ability of the kidney to produce a concentrated urine, since some physiologists held this to be a key indicator of its "power." As other workers added measurements of dye excretion and "urea loads," the term "renal insufficiency" entered the language of Bright's Disease.[18] The insufficient kidney lacked normal power and reserve to deal with an increasing demand to excrete substances. Further weakening later became known as renal failure, which meant frank retention of urea and those other waste materials usually discharged by the renal filters. These new names indicated the early twentieth-century enthusiasm for trying to understand disease in terms of what an injured organ could or could not do rather than how it looked. "Acute renal failure" and "chronic renal failure" continue in use as of when I write this, though as will be seen later, a movement of the 1990s centered in the United States sought, with considerable success, to banish the term "chronic renal failure" in favor of "chronic kidney disease."

The French physiologist Fernand Widal (1862–1929) divided Bright's Disease into a type in which salt retention dominates and thus the patient shows mainly edema, since salt "holds" water; and a type in which urea retention dominates and the patient shows toxicity from such retained solutes. A third type he linked to the development of arterial hypertension.[19] Although this proposed functional classification did not supplant the structural schemes available, Widal's work did induce succeeding clinicians and physiologists to at least think more physiologically and to separate salt retention and nitrogen retention in their minds and in their therapeutics. Following Widal's proposals, restriction of salt in the diet came into use for reducing or preventing edema.

Thus, as some physicians of the twentieth century became experts in generalized kidney disease (Bright's Disease), they analyzed it in two ways. One way sought to establish types, a classification, based on visible appearances of the diseased kidney structure viewed under the microscope. The other was to measure the injured kidney's ability to function, do its job, particularly its capacity to excrete bodily wastes such as urea. These two approaches (which might also be termed structural and physiological) are by no means mutually exclusive, and the care of the patient has required both. As will be seen later in the book, however, when renal function reaches a point of extreme deterioration, the pathological category matters little.

PUTTING IT ALL TOGETHER: THOMAS ADDIS, MD

Thomas Addis represents one of several figures who brought together the structural and functional ways of viewing renal disease. Addis was a Scottish physician with sound chemical training hired as a young man by the new Stanford University School of Medicine in 1911.[20] There he took up in the clinic and in the laboratory a lifelong study of Bright's Disease. Through intense and sustained work with patients and in the rat laboratory, he became one of the first comprehensive authorities on renal disease in the twentieth century. He titled his monumental book of 1931 (with pathologist Jean Oliver) *The Renal Lesion in Bright's Disease*. A lavishly illustrated work of clinical-pathological correlation based on autopsy but including many results from the laboratory, in form and purpose it recalled Richard Bright's *Reports of Medical Cases* of one hundred years earlier. By "renal lesion" he meant both the type of disordered structure *and* the amount of lost function. His three-component scheme for the pathologic classification of Bright's Disease achieved its usefulness, Addis believed, from its direct linkage with his method of standardizing and quantifying the urine sediment examination. That is, in the 1920s he devised a standardized technique for counting the number of casts and cells in a urine sample examined microscopically. A certain count of red cells, for example, might suggest the hemorrhagic form of Bright's Disease (glomerulonephritis), whereas a dominance of casts favored the degenerative type. This test became known as the Addis Count and attained widespread use. It was a way of modernizing for the era of laboratory medicine a traditional diagnostic aid—microscopic examination of the urine—by transforming it into a value expressed quantitatively.

Addis wanted to add to the structural diagnosis—which pathological form of Bright's Disease does this person have?—a functional diagnosis: how much of the kidneys' primary job can they still carry out for the "nephritic" patient, as he or she was now sometimes referred to? Since by then it was long held that the kidneys are responsible for eliminating nitrogenous wastes (breakdown products of protein) from the body, like his predecessors he focused on urea, by the 1920s easily quantified in urine and blood samples. Aware that the simple concentration of urea in the blood can vary a good deal in healthy persons, he devised a more sophisticated indicator using both blood and urine values, which he called the "urea ratio." It showed the kidneys' ability to excrete urea at a given level of blood urea and could be expressed as a percentage of expected normal. Thus he would conceive that a patient with a certain decreased urea ratio had "69% of renal tissue proper for her size." Even when using such a numerical indicator, Addis still envisioned actual renal "mass," a mark of his upbringing in an era of medicine whose bedrock was still pathology.

Later in his career, in the 1940s, Addis abandoned the urea ratio and adopted the simple concentration of creatinine in the blood as his indication of remaining renal function, though he was not the first to do so.[21] The use of the blood creatinine as the single most critical indicator of renal well-being found universal acceptance in the period after World War II and continues into the twenty-first century. Creatinine, a harmless product of muscle cells, finds its way into the blood, then is filtered out through the kidneys. It happens that it rises in the blood in exact proportion to the decrease in renal function, meaning here decrease in filtration of solutes (waste products). Also, fairly simple techniques have allowed its measurement in a small sample of blood. An elevated creatinine value in a patient came to *be* "renal failure."

For specialists in renal medicine of the late twentieth century, it would no longer literally call to mind an anatomic image of shrunken renal tissue, as did the urea ratio for Addis, who frequently saw such kidneys at autopsies. But the *number,* the creatinine concentration expressed usually as milligrams in 100 milliliters of blood, would acquire an ominous power, as had the *name* "Bright's Disease" in the nineteenth century. The "normal range" is up to about 1.5. Values of 2 or 3 tell of a very substantial loss of the kidney's critical excretory capacity, but persons with chronic renal disease with such readings don't have symptoms. A preventive regimen of diet and drugs will be prescribed. A creatinine value of 6 or 7, however, raises alarm: it heralds the imminent need for more drastic measures, such as dialysis treatment or kidney transplantation. In the more recent care of chronic Bright's Disease (called something else, of course, by the 1940s), both physician and the knowledgeable patient endure some level of anxiety awaiting the results of the next "chemistry panel" with its value for the creatinine. Indeed, during the afternoon when I worked on this very paragraph, a call from my clinical office reported creatinine values for two of my outpatients. Both were a bit higher than the readings at their last visit (a rising creatinine, despite their best efforts and mine!). Hearing these numbers still provided me some minutes of real unease, even after decades of practice. And the worry will be greater for the patients and their families.

Chronic Bright's Disease, by whatever name, in fact does tend to progress: once the kidney has suffered some episode of destructive disease, even if that inciting event has passed entirely, kidney size and function tend to slowly shrink away, usually over a period of years. This phenomenon, once it was clearly appreciated, maintained the grim reputation of Bright's Disease. Thomas Addis took this seemingly inevitable deterioration to be the dominant challenge and tried to understand it through the laboratory by creating rat "models" of impaired kidneys. After an immense amount of study, he concluded that once some of the kidneys' nephrons have been destroyed by disease, the remaining nephrons (each human kidney comprises about 800,000 individual units) try to compensate by increasing their action, but then tend gradually to "burn out" from overwork.[22] A downhill spiral ensues, which could only lead to death before measures became available (well after Addis's time) to replace kidney function, namely, dialysis and transplantation.

Addis further concluded that the main work of the kidneys was excreting urea in a concentrated form. Since the need to excrete urea arises from the eating of protein, urea being its main metabolic waste product, Addis theorized that the remaining kidney structure (the surviving, overworking nephrons) could be "rested," and protected from overwork injury, by reducing dietary protein. He proved that this worked in his rats and implemented the low-protein diet in a meticulous way in his clinical practice at San Francisco (the location of Stanford University School of Medicine in Addis's time). This approach fit the therapeutics of the 1920s and 1930s, a period when dietetics formed a critical part of management of diabetes, ulcer, typhoid fever, gout, bowel disorders, and all manner of ailments. In those decades, a hospital nutrition manual could display over fifty different diets that might be prescribed. Some practitioners with a special interest in the treatment of albuminuric renal disease held viewpoints entirely different from Addis's, however, and gave high-protein diets. Their notion was to replace protein lost through the urine and to overall "strengthen" the kidneys. They reserved the low-protein diet for those individuals whose blood tests already showed high amounts of retained nitrogenous substances such as urea.[23]

Addis seems to have succeeded in keeping his patients on the protein-restricted, and sometimes salt-limited, diets for years at a time because of his direct participation in their care, his willingness to engage the patient as an ally, and his reliance on a team. Using the term "glomerular nephritis" rather than "Bright's Disease," he wrote: "The conclusion drawn from our experience is that a successful conjunction of theory and practice in dietetics of glomerular nephritis requires the simultaneous collaboration of at least four people, i.e., the patient, the laboratory technician, the doctor, and the dietician. I believe it is not only necessary for these four to be working at the same time, they must also be in the same room, for each one has necessary objective facts to present, and it is in the conversation of these four people, that the fusion of theory and practice is obtained."[24]

Addis was a left-leaning progressive—egalitarian, strongly anti-Fascist, and intensely interested in the social and economic context of medicine and of his own patients. Bright's Disease afforded him the opportunity to forge his physiological and social beliefs into a therapeutic environment, centered on the ancient pathways of dietetics and implemented by a community of active participants. Addis believed that the person carrying out the tedious assays for protein in the urine, or urea in the plasma, must literally *see* that there is a patient involved in the enterprise. Similarly, the patient should appreciate the role of the laboratory workers. Other chronic maladies might have served nearly as well, but chronic proteinuric kidney disease perfectly fit Addis's way of mixing research with practical care, as it had done for Richard Bright.

The investigation and treatment of Bright's Disease as Addis chose to do it, embracing the idea of the team or "group," as he liked to call it, nicely suited as well his socialist worldview.

Of course, there were other physicians and scientists exploring Bright's Disease during the first half of the twentieth century, both in Europe and the United States. Another American worker (and friend of Tom Addis) was Donald D. Van Slyke (1883–1971), chemist at the Hospital of the Rockefeller Institute for Medical Research. "Rounding" over many years with physicians of the hospital, Van Slyke became conversant with the clinical attributes and treatment of kidney disease. His ingenious analytical device (the "Van Slyke apparatus") and theoretical powers led to new understandings of the variability of renal filtration in different circumstances and of the kidney's role in regulating the balance of acids and alkali in blood. Van Slyke and his colleagues also contributed a major publication correlating the clinical, pathological, and chemical findings for a series of patients with kidney disease.[25] That Van Slyke, a chemist, could attain recognition as one of the preeminent authorities on Bright's Disease indicates the standing of the laboratory within renal medicine (and medicine more generally) by the 1920s.

The attention to Addis and Van Slyke and the shift in location within these last few pages to the United States represent more than mere chauvinism. To be sure, Franz Volhard of Germany remained a master of renal medicine during the years between World War I and World War II, and articles on the function and diseases of the kidneys continued to appear in the German medical journals. By the mid-1930s, Robert Platt (1900–1978) of Great Britain attained standing for his work in kidney disease and hypertension.[26] But this was the time when medical research in the United States came of age. The movement for reform of American medical education, beginning in the late 1870s, closed weak colleges and transformed the stronger university schools, particularly encouraging the ideology of research. Philanthropic foundations, the products of enormous aggregations of money gained through industrial capitalism—mostly oil, steel, and railroads—paid for the bettering of U.S. schools of medicine and for much of the burgeoning medical research. Donald Van Slyke worked at the

Hospital of the Rockefeller Institute, America's first well-funded medical research establishment, built and sustained, of course, by the Rockefellers. Tom Addis spent a year with Van Slyke at the institute in 1928 and later obtained grants from other Rockefeller programs. Two nonphysician scientists who made major contributions to renal physiology, A. Newton Richards (1876–1966) of the University of Pennsylvania, and Homer W. Smith (1895–1962) at New York University, enjoyed long-term financial support from the Commonwealth Fund, which virtually "adopted" the kidney as its favorite organ. The physiologic contributions of Richards and Smith, beginning in the 1930s, further identified the United States as the new center for the study of the kidney and its diseases. Both collaborated with clinicians, and the revered Homer Smith virtually created a new language for renal physiology in health and disease.[27]

On whatever continent, disease of the kidneys since the 1820s has provided fruitful and seemingly inexhaustible opportunities for medical study, whether descriptive—at the bedside, autopsy table, or microscope; or chemical—carried out in the laboratory. Its classification continues to evolve and expand. The kidney's dominant role in regulating the fine chemical composition of the blood (and entire body for that matter) has meant that renal diseases produce a myriad of consequences capable of quantitative exploration.[28] Thus there existed several pathways for studying the normal and diseased kidney. Furthermore, vital statistics showed Bright's Disease (or "nephritis") to have been, in the United States, between the fourth and sixth most common cause of death during the period 1900 to 1940.[29] It is not surprising that foundations were willing to pay for renal research, especially in forward-looking laboratories.

This chapter will conclude by further illustrating some of the manifestations of Bright's Disease, and one form of treatment in the mid-twentieth century, with another patient's story.

THOMAS ADDIS SHARES A PATIENT

In March of 1941, a prominent theoretical chemist from California visited New York City to receive an award and offer a lecture. The event took place at the then illustrious Hotel Pennsylvania. The chemist held the reputation for lively speech-making, but something seemed amiss: his voice sounded dull, and his demeanor lacked energy. Those sitting close to the podium could discern that his face looked puffy, and he had in fact awakened that day with his eyes swollen shut. He revealed to some friends the next evening that he had felt worn out for some weeks yet had gained about twenty pounds of weight and had a hard time fitting into his shoes. Some physician friends arranged for a rapid workup (examination and testing) at the Hospital of the Rockefeller Institute, under the direction of cardiologist Alfred E. Cohn. The tests revealed 12 grams of protein per liter of urine, a very large amount. The Rockefeller Hospital chemist and expert on all things renal, Donald Van Slyke, easily concluded that the visiting scientist was "suffering from some form of nephritis," though when the man and his wife heard the news, the label was probably "Bright's Disease." Cohn promptly wrote to his friend Tom Addis in San Francisco, hoping he could look after the patient—the chemist was now, suddenly, a patient—on his return to California.

On the long train ride home, worry prevailed in the couple's compartment: the chemist recalled that his grandfather on his father's side had died from some sort of kidney disease. Upon arriving home, he read up on renal ailments, and hardly found encouragement. Though still more tired than usual, and edematous, he chose to dismiss worry as much as he could through a return to work, or as much as his own doctor would allow. The local physician advised "rest," so some new grant proposals and other writing were accomplished in bed. Further examination of the urine confirmed heavy albuminuria and also showed some granular casts. The patient interrupted his odd combination of bed rest and work long enough to have two abscessed teeth extracted; this may have been scheduled anyway, or it might have been thought that the smoldering infection could somehow have brought on the nephritis, a familiar idea of the time. Some puffiness of the patient's hands, face, and feet continued, and he had the peculiar sensation that his tongue felt "thick."

The patient, Linus Pauling (1901–1994), survived his renal disease to become recognized as one of the most important scientists of the twentieth century, twice a Nobel Laureate (first for Chemistry, later the Peace Prize for his antinuclear activism).[30] Thomas Addis supervised the care of Pauling's "nephritis" (the general category of his kidney disorder would now be called nephrotic syndrome), though it was implemented, and perfectly so, by Mrs. Pauling. Ava Helen Pauling (1903–1981) had studied home economics in college and through the early part of her life devoted her considerable energy and intelligence to running the Pauling household and raising the couple's four children, while her husband grew his career. "Home economics" was the name given beginning in the early twentieth century to the study and teaching of "scientific" domestic management in colleges and universities. It included nutrition and cooking. Later, Ava Helen Pauling would, with her husband and through her own works, become a forceful voice for peace and human rights. But for some years beginning in March of 1941, she directed her talents to the preparation of low-protein meals, as specified within 5-gram increments by Tom Addis. The diet at first also had to contain the least possible salt, since Addis believed that sick kidneys might be saved, or at least their working life prolonged, by reducing the "work" of excreting the nitrogenous waste products of protein. The salt restriction aimed at lessening the edema. Much of the communication about the diet and other aspects of management—mostly between Addis and Ava Helen—occurred through letters, since the Paulings were in Pasadena (where Linus worked at the California Institute of Technology) and Addis was in San Francisco. Pauling did visit Addis's clinic a few times each year.

Pauling gave up all forms of meat, though he ate an occasional egg at breakfast. A typical lunch included some macaroni or potato, salad, and fruit. Supper on January 2, 1942, was representative: milk, potatoes, spinach, lemon pie, and some cream: 23 grams of protein, making 49 grams for the day with breakfast and lunch. Mrs. Pauling calculated and recorded the content of protein for every part of every meal.[31] This dietary astringency produced psychological as well as physiological effects. In a letter to Tom Addis from May 20, 1941, Ava Helen wrote the following: "I asked him [Linus] what his thoughts were the other day and he said, 'Oh, turtle soup, chicken[,] bacon.' So you see the poets were all together wrong about the 'far-away' look in a man's eye. I've often suspected as much."[32] In July of 1941, Mrs. Pauling arranged for an exact analysis of the constituents of a 1-inch cube of Mexican Jack cheese, which Linus enjoyed. Finding its protein and salt content minimal, she permitted him one such portion daily. This modification arose when the Paulings were in Chicago during a wretchedly hot July. Ava Helen astutely raised the salt content of her partner's diet, knowing he would lose much through sweat. In fact, his remaining edema vanished in Chicago—"it has been evaporated by this fiendish weather."[33] The sweating regimen does work for some dropsies.

By April and May, Pauling already had been feeling better—stronger, less swollen, in a better mood, his ambition returning. His lecturing grew sharper, and his ability to concentrate improved. But, as typical with Bright's Disease or its successors in name, "there are fluctuations. Some days better than others."[34] Pauling's local physician reported to Addis by letter in late May that the patient still showed some edema of the legs and over the lower back and lost 4 to 9 grams of protein in the urine each day.[35] Dr. McMillan agreed that Pauling's frame of mind was much improved; he was recovering at least from the shock of the diagnosis of Bright's Disease. In the middle of June 1941, Pauling reported directly to Addis that he had been "feeling well, working steadily at my writing, and not worrying about anything."[36] He also had been running protein analyses on his own urine, not trusting the results of his local physician! He found a rather high rate of protein loss, with a heavier spillage during the day than overnight. A note obviously added later to the bottom of one sheet of calculations in Pauling's laboratory books says, "About this time Dr. Addis told me to stop analyzing my own urine."[37]

Thomas Addis showed an eager interest in the lives and individuality of his patients, including Linus Pauling, who became a close friend, as did Mrs. Pauling.[38] Yet his approach as a doctor, at least for Pauling, reveals a deep strand of what has come to be known as medical paternalism. In letters to Ava Helen, Addis repeatedly urged that Linus remain, in relation to his Bright's Disease, "wholly passive." He should know "that everything possible is being done and [should be] forgetting the matter altogether." "We finally decided to make you the doctor," Addis told Ava Helen, and the two of them would look after Linus's kidneys. "You are his doctor," Addis repeated in another letter, pleased with the notion. "Let him forget all about it."[39] Pauling obviously cannot forget about his illness when doing assays of his own urinary protein, so Addis ordered him to desist. Because of Pauling's special expertise, however, Addis could not refrain from sharing with the chemist his concept of renal work, and Pauling enthusiastically recalculated some of Addis's data and commented on the theory. But Addis eventually apologized for thus making the patient too cognizant of the disease. "I can't help bothering you with these questions. But it is bad. You should forget all this. You're in fine shape. Did I tell you how low your plasma urea went—8.8 mgs for 100 cc!"[40]

The physician wanted Pauling to forget his illness not only to reduce anxiety and distress but to serve a higher need: Pauling must be able to "free himself for his work."[41] For Tom Addis, the objective of medical care for the person with a chronic disease, and the mark of its success or failure, was not so much length of survival, or degree of feeling well, but a *man's ability to go to work.* In *Glomerular Nephritis* Addis narrated the course of another, unnamed scientist, a young university physicist who had become "an essential element in the life of a group," a working laboratory group similar to Addis's. The "social importance of our patient's life is very obvious," wrote Addis, who no doubt thought the same about Pauling, "but . . . it is true of the lives of all patients. It is our job to do our best to keep them on the firing line to the very last gasp."[42] Of course, the Stanford renal specialist who put in endless hours in the clinic and rat lab could easily identify with other scientists. But preserved notes from his practice show constant attention to the *work*—or lack of it—of patients such as "P.H.," a young man who strived to find and keep employment during the Depression while also enduring Bright's Disease and a 45-gram protein diet. P.H. drove a taxi, clerked in a cigar store, and in desperation panned for gold.[43]

I don't know if any of Addis's patients were women who worked outside their home, and if so, whether he also defined them in terms of their work. (Several women scientists did work in his laboratory, and not only as technologists; and Addis's wife served as his dietician.) He readily enrolled Mrs. Linus Pauling as nutritionist, cook, and eventually as deputy "doctor," subservient employment in the service of keeping her husband active at his job. Her letters to Addis show that Ava Helen took pride in her dietary expertise and ability to foresee the need for adjustments and to implement them independently. Once it became clear that Linus's laboratory results were showing consistently decreasing amounts of proteinuria, she, understandably, felt a confidence that Linus would eventually recover entirely. The more cautious Addis allowed that some residual signs of the disease might persist indefinitely, though not enough to have a "bearing on length of life or capacity for work."[44]

The male physicians of the nineteenth and early twentieth centuries so far encountered at some length in this book—Richard Bright, James Tyson, William Osler, Thomas Addis—all put in prodigious amounts of time working: they mixed practice, research of some sort, teaching, voluminous writing, and organizational work. They embodied two related, and by now tiresome, phrases—"Protestant work ethic" and "workaholic." By their day, the industrial age had come to virtually equate a man with his work. William Osler, though he much valued friendships and literature, taught that "happiness lies in the absorption in some vocation which satisfied the soul."[45] Recall that Bright—whose second wife, Eliza, often complained that he worked too much—included the occupations of his Guy's Hospital patients in his case narratives, often as the only personal detail other than drinking habits.[46] And it was the ability to resume and continue work as a bookbinder that served as the primary marker of the clinical well-being of Bright's office patient described in chapter 3. The patrician Philadelphia physician, physiologist, and novelist S. Weir Mitchell, in an essay recalling with pleasure his own time of convalescence from a bout of grave illness (not a kidney disease), referred to "the long road towards working health." That is, for Mitchell, a return to work signifies, or perhaps *is*, the return to something called "health."[47] Historian Sheila Rothman has described how young men with consumptive symptoms wrote in agony not so much of the expectation of a shortened life but rather of the regret in giving up particular occupational plans.[48]

After the first few months of his Bright's Disease, Linus Pauling never felt so ill as to leave his work altogether. He, his wife, and his physician measured his improvement in several ways: disappearance of the dropsy, greater strength and energy, trends toward the normal in laboratory measurements, and greater vitality at the job, especially when lecturing. Within about four years of its onset, Pauling's kidney disease, obviously a nonfatal variety, had resolved. Following Addis's theory and his advice, he stayed on the low-protein diet for a total of fourteen years. He lived to the age of ninety-three, actively working most of that time, in science, peace advocacy, and later, promoting the value of vitamin C.[49] By the time the world lost this idiosyncratic genius in 1994, Addis's theory and the low-protein diet for renal disease had all but vanished for several decades, and then attracted a new wave of interest as chronic renal disease came to seem epidemic in the 1980s. Beginning in the 1960s, it was hemodialysis, the "artificial kidney," not the low-protein diet, that medicine offered to keep alive many persons with otherwise fatal renal failure. They were alive but by no means always out "on the firing line" of work and life.

⟞☙⟝

A Later Perspective

We will have more to say about the evolving categorization and terminology of what was once Bright's Disease in the remaining chapters, and have already pointed out in the preceding text some concepts that have proved durable. "Acute hemorrhagic Bright's Disease" became "acute glomerulonephritis," and this increasingly became understood as an inflammatory process within the glomerular capillary tuft created by some disordered immunological reaction—that is, the body's immune system, rather than some external toxin or microbe, comes to attack the glomerulus. In its fullest, most expressive form, the disease causes flank pain, blood in the urine accompanied by protein and casts, salt and fluid retention (edema), and sometimes failure of kidney function, usually transient. In its most severe form, it can lead to uremia, which will be recalled as the symptom complex caused by failure of renal excretory function, including nausea, vomiting, chest pains, itching, muscle twitching, and even convulsions and coma. As we have noted, the form of acute glomerulonephritis longest recognized, referred to still as poststreptococcal, is triggered by a streptococcal infection of the throat or skin but clearly represents some "secondary" immune response, not a "primary" streptococcal invasion of the kidney.

Another type of glomerulonephritis (there are many), unrecognized until the 1960s and the advent of kidney biopsy (introduced in chapter 5), is known as IgA nephropathy, or immunoglobulin A nephropathy. Immunoglobulin A denotes one type of antibody. Antibodies are the protein substances manufactured by specialized cells that bind to and "neutralize" potentially injurious microscopic objects that have entered the body, such as viruses, bacteria, or pollen. The primary symptom of IgA nephropathy is bleeding into the urine, and it sometimes occurs in association with sore throats, like poststreptococcal glomerulonephritis. IgA nephropathy (first called Berger's Disease after a French pathologist who described it) is caused by some poorly understood failure of normal regulation of that part of the antibody-producing system of the human body which is, in part, located in the smooth "mucosal" linings of the air passages, throat, and intestines. It is now believed that IgA nephropathy is the most common form of glomerulonephritis in the world; fortunately, it does not commonly lead to progressive loss of kidney function. There is no way to know if IgA nephropathy existed in the nineteenth century.

As pointed out earlier in this volume, a functional category of kidney disease marked by extreme loss of albumin into the urine through "leaky" glomeruli came to be known as nephrotic syndrome, a term still used. Its hallmark is dropsy, or edema, and of course it would include some cases previously included with Bright's Disease. The "chronic parenchymatous nephritis" of Osler, the "nephroses" of Volhard and Fahr, and Addis's "degenerative Bright's disease" probably included a variety of renal disorders centered in the glomeruli that created the complex of findings known later as nephrotic syndrome. Nephrologists and pathologists now apply to nephrotic syndrome a very refined categorization scheme based on conventional and electron microscopy. The names for the specific disorders, however, remain cumbersome and strange—"membranous nephropathy," or "focal segmental glomerulosclerosis," for example. "Amyloidosis" remains in use as the name for a set of rare glomerular diseases that produce nephrotic syndrome, which are caused by the deposition in the filtering membranes of one or another poorly soluble protein. Some types of amyloidosis of the kidney are familial; others result from overstimulation of the immune system.

Finally, we have the "nephroscleroses" of Volhard and Fahr and "arteriosclerotic Bright's Disease" of Addis. At least to some extent, these correlate with the now very common form of renal injury caused by high blood pressure, or hypertension. Hypertensive renal disease has become a dominant cause of complete loss of kidney function, particularly among persons of color. It has become increasingly apparent as well that given some other basis for chronic kidney disease (e.g., diabetes), reduction of elevated blood pressure counts as one of the most important measures to slow worsening of the disorder.

Although this book centers on medicine and patients in the West, dropsy / Bright's Disease / nephrotic syndrome / glomerulonephritis has afflicted huge numbers of people in the tropics, especially Africa. Through complex immunologic mechanisms, a secondary renal disease often follows infections with parasites such as malaria, trypanosomiasis, schistosomiasis, and filariasis. Poverty and the disruptions caused by civil wars limit eradication programs and infestation rates soar. The incidence of proteinuric renal disease and kidney failure similarly rises.[50] Glomerular disease can also occur as a complication of infection with certain of the hepatitis viruses and the human immunodeficiency virus (HIV), further adding to the enormous amount of kidney disease in the developing world, and in the West as well.

What about making the diagnosis of renal disease? Nephrologists and sometimes other physicians still use the microscope to examine the urine, and the presence of casts still holds meaning. Thomas Addis's quantitative count of casts and cells in the urine has, however, disappeared from use. As pointed out in the main text of this chapter, measurement of blood creatinine continues in widespread use to assess the overall amount of filtering capacity that remains in a person with kidney disease. We still pay some attention to the urea content of blood, though to some extent the urea value in today's laboratory printout represents an historical artifact, a continuation from earlier times that no one has thought to shut off.

We used Thomas Addis's contributions to summarize an approach to Bright's Disease (again, meaning mainly chronic, protein-losing kidney disease) as of the early 1940s, a time just preceding an enormous expansion of scientific research and technology within medicine. Addis was, admittedly, somewhat idiosyncratic in his beliefs, and certainly in his politics and manner of running his practice and research laboratory. His way of understanding the inherently progressive nature of many sorts of kidney disease (the propensity for the filtering capacity and other functions to slowly worsen over time) in terms of the organ work and rest did not gain wide acceptance in his day. But, as we will see in chapter 9, a reformulation of Addis's theory, or at least a concept similar to it, arose in the 1980s to invigorate new efforts to preserve the functioning of diseased kidneys. Within debates about how to do this, the low-protein meal was back on the table, not in the setting of Addis's precise rendering for a few, but rather as the subject of large "controlled trials," enrolling hundreds. The exact role of the low-protein diet in trying to slow progression of chronic renal disease remains unsettled as this is written. There exists agreement, however, that some protein restriction in the diet (particularly animal-based protein) will at least delay and lessen the symptoms of uremia.

Linus Pauling's renal disease, marked by severe albuminuria and edema but not uremia, would fall into the current broad category of "nephrotic syndrome." He may have had the particular disorder called membranous nephropathy (mentioned above), an indolent process known sometimes to resolve with treatment, or on its own, or a similar condition called minimal change disease, though this tends to occur mainly in children (it was once known as childhood nephrotic syndrome). There is, of course, no way to know with any certainty what specific pathological subtype afflicted Pauling or whether the low-protein diet was curative.

CHAPTER FIVE

Renal Shutdown, a Needle, and the End of Bright's Disease

—⊰⊱⊱—

Thomas Addis's *Glomerular Nephritis: Diagnosis and Treatment,* a summative statement of his theory and practice, appeared in 1948. He had used "Bright's Disease" in the title of his 1931 book, but that term was out of date by 1948. So was publishing new medical ideas in a book: by that time, researchers placed their findings in the weekly or monthly medical journals. For this reason and others, Addis's concepts of kidney disease and its dietary treatment would sink into obscurity for many years.[1] Also in 1948, an article in a monthly journal of internal medicine included the following case report. In early January of that year, "E.R.," an indigent twenty-five-year-old single woman in New York City was raped. When her next menstruation failed to occur, no doubt confirming her most awful fears, she inserted five "sublimate of mercury" tablets into the vagina in order to induce abortion, as reported in the article, which owned the strange title "Experience with the Kolff Artificial Kidney."[2] "Sublimate of mercury" was an old term for mercuric chloride, or mercuric bichloride, a material once widely available as an "antiseptic" and also used for some ill-defined medicinal purposes. Another of the substance's names, "corrosive sublimate," more than hints at its properties: over several hundred years it accumulated a baneful history of application in homicide and suicide—and, in desperation, as an agent to induce abortion. None of the United States allowed abortion in 1948, though no doubt those Americans more affluent than the subject of this case could find a less hazardous solution than her solitary and miserable resort.

Soon the young woman was wretchedly ill with abdominal pain, bloody diarrhea, vomiting, and profuse vaginal bleeding. She was admitted to the gynecological service of one New York hospital, then was transferred to Mount Sinai Hospital. Mount Sinai had been founded in the nineteenth century primarily to offer accommodation to Jewish physicians, who usually could not gain clinical privileges at the better hospitals in American cities. It matured into an internationally known center of medical research and innovation while still offering charity care to all who showed up at its doors. Mount Sinai accepted the woman in transfer to its internal medicine service because as part of her toxic illness, her kidneys had stopped functioning (a "medical" more than "gynecological" complication). As urine production ceased altogether, urea, creatinine, and other substances rapidly accumulated in her blood. Mount Sinai had recently acquired a remarkable new device, the "artificial kidney," which, it was thought, might prove helpful in treating exactly this complication.

The physicians trying out the novel apparatus at Mount Sinai Hospital (as listed in their publication) were Alfred P. Fishman, Irving G. Kroop, H. Evans Leiter, and Abraham Hyman, but it was really Drs. Fishman and Kroop, both young men, who did the work. On arrival, they wrote, the woman looked "poorly developed, poorly nourished" (a statement about "poorly developed" versus "well-developed," and "-nourished," was by then the stereotypic beginning of a case presentation and continues as such in some medical teaching settings today). She was "semicomatose . . . vomiting coffee-ground material [partly-digested blood] and blood was oozing from her mouth and gums. She looked pale and her face was edematous." The tongue and mouth were inflamed, and the genitalia were also red, swollen, and "covered with exudates." Her blood pressure was surprisingly well maintained. There is no statement about whether she could talk at this point, and if so, what she tried to say; probably she could not. She was treated with BAL (British anti-Lewisite, a very odd name for a medication, now known as dimercaprol, an agent to inactivate and remove mercury). She also received penicillin and intravenous fluids. Methods to produce penicillin in large quantity had been devised during World War II, so its use for this woman in 1948 (to prevent complicating infection) marked her treatment as entirely up to date, even before the artificial kidney was deployed.

"At 11 p.m. on the day of admission," reads the case narrative, one of six in the article, "treatment with the artificial kidney was started and was continued for six hours. . . . All observers agreed that she improved markedly during this time. She became less restless, better oriented, and was able to request and retain oral fluids." The authors of the article then present, within the text and graphically, a great amount of laboratory data that documents the effectiveness of the machine in removing retained urea and chloride from the patient's blood and tissues. But it is the simple testimony of witnesses to this historic therapeutic event to which the writers appeal in order to convince the reader that the artificial kidney worked—"all observers agreed" that she got better. This continues a rhetorical device in science going back to the seventeenth century and the Royal Society, by which specified on-site witnesses stand in for the reader, who of course could not be in the laboratory to see the experiment.[3] The patient became better "oriented," presumably a good thing, unless perhaps she could now better remember the occurrence that had begun her series of crises. Again, in the ritual objectified wording of such case reports (of the sort that I too once employed) "she was able to request and retain oral fluids." Did she "request" in English or Spanish? Did she ask for coffee, apple juice, cola?

The managing physicians carefully prescribed a diet rich in calories but containing no protein, and a variety of fluids containing sodium bicarbonate and sodium chloride, the amounts determined by blood measurements. Over the week following the session with the artificial kidney, a gradual reappearance of urinary flow indicated that her own injured kidneys had begun to recover. The amount of fluid leaving her as urine and through the skin and lungs did not yet match the fluids she took in, and some mild edema of the face and legs occurred. She continued to recover, however, and the various areas eroded by the corrosive sublimate were healing well. But on the twelfth day of hospitalization, following menstruation, she unexpectedly became agitated and "hypomanic," with paranoid delusions and hallucinations "centered around the events which had initiated the present illness." Having benefited maximally from the sophisticated therapeutics at Mount Sinai, she was sent to a third facility, the Rockland State Hospital in Orangeburg, New York, for psychiatric care, reputedly the setting for a novel and film of the 1940s titled *The Snake Pit*.[4] She was still there in March of 1948, but her renal blood tests measured then were virtually normal.

At this point, her story as recorded in the article ends, a succès d'estime of sorts, a qualified victory for the revolutionary therapy. The machine, by substituting briefly for her own damaged kidneys, had very likely deferred death from uremia long enough for her body, including her own filters, to heal. Her mind, however, when we leave E.R., had not been cleansed of "the events which had initiated the present illness." She had to be sent from the modern home of the artificial organ to a state hospital for the insane, a holdover from the nineteenth century. Her medical saga comprised three chapters at three hospitals—she was another case of botched abortion when on the gynecological service of the first (unnamed) hospital; at Mount Sinai she was "acute toxic nephrosis," managed successfully with physiologically guided diet and fluids and a remarkable new machine; at Rockland she was insane, and we don't know the nature of her care.

I do not intend to imply that her team of physicians and other caregivers (she must have obligated a huge amount of nursing work) at Mount Sinai thought only about the woman's blood tests or saw her as merely a suitable subject for the new treatment. The physicians, all men, had girlfriends, wives, perhaps daughters. They probably felt very badly about her plight, joyous when she turned the corner, stunned and disappointed when the course took the unexpected turn toward madness. Quite likely they perceived the irony and paradox of the story they told, one whose lesson would be increasingly demonstrated in twentieth-century hospitals: a technological success does not always predict a restoration to well-being.

Just as Richard Bright, by all accounts a compassionate man, presented his first readers with color plates of kidneys and clinical details more than human stories, so was it the job of the authors of "Experience with the Kolff Artificial Kidney" (regardless of what their feelings might have been) to present dispassionately, as convention required, their experience with the Kolff artificial kidney. Bright's *Reports of Medical Cases* of 1827 and this article about the new kidney machine 120 years later display similar rules about medical case-telling, but each typified its medical era and presented what seemed new and important. For Bright, it was the relationship of proteinuria to particular appearances of the kidney at autopsy; for the authors of 1948, it was the use and performance of a kidney machine. Drs. Fishman and Kroop did include one illustration, which they captioned "the artificial kidney in use" (not reproduced here). It is cropped to show the rotating-drum machine centered in and occupying most of the image; only part of the left arm of the patient can be seen at the edge, blood lines connected. The machine, the real subject of the article, takes center stage. Of course, the authors may have made this choice in part to preserve confidentiality.

This was the story of the first successful use of hemodialysis—the artificial kidney—in the United States, though not at all the first in the world. In fact, the machine itself was sent to New York by its inventor, Willem Kolff (b. 1911), a Dutch physician who would soon emigrate and become part of America's explosive postwar dominance in biomedicine. The inventive Canadian surgeon Gordon Murray (1894–1976) had carried out the first dialysis in North America in 1946 in Toronto, using an artificial kidney of his own design though based on the same principles as that of Kolff. As it happens, that first Canadian patient treated with dialysis was also a young woman with sudden kidney failure caused by a self-induced abortion.[5]

The artificial kidney, or hemodialyzer, conveys the patient's blood outside the body and through a filter made of a membranous cellophane-like material that allows removal of retained substances and also a quantity of water from the blood but not the loss of the various blood cells and proteins. The Kolff machine arrayed tubing of actual cellophane (cellulose acetate, then in use as a sausage casing!) around a large rotating wooden drum set in a "bath" of fluid designed to attract from the blood those solutes in need of removal. The care of the Mount Sinai patient with mercuric bichloride poisoning using this large machine certainly approached the heroic: the authors even mention that the treatment commenced at eleven at night. They concluded, however, with attractive modesty, that "the artificial kidney may have provided additional time for spontaneous improvement to occur," referring to the return of renal function.[6] These physicians used a new device to treat a patient with a more or less "new" kidney disease, or at least a newly recognized concept in medicine—reversible "acute renal failure." We will, of course, return to the story of the artificial kidney later, a story still characterized by incomplete fulfillment. But here we will further introduce this new disorder, or really set of related disorders.

ACUTE RENAL FAILURE

In a lengthy article from 1953 titled "The Clinical Course of Acute Renal Failure," Boston physicians Roy C. Swann and John P. Merrill wrote: "During the past ten years a new concept of acute reversible renal failure has emerged. This concept has provided a common understanding of several previously apparently unrelated renal disorders and has resulted in a profound change in the therapeutic approach to acute oliguria."[7]

John P. Merrill (1917–1986) of Boston would become an American leader in developing the use of hemodialysis (which I will use synonymously with "artificial kidney") and kidney transplantation. "Oliguria" refers to a very much decreased production of urine, an amount so little that even with maximal concentration a typical daily load of urinary waste substances could not be discharged in it. Oliguria usually signifies a sudden cessation of renal function. Although Swann and Merrill wrote that the concept of acute renal failure "emerged," as if it were a new being that crept from obscurity into medical view, one might alternatively say that interested clinicians fashioned a coherent model out of a variety of similar clinical observations described in medical journals during the 1930s and 1940s. To some extent they were restoring a disease concept that was not truly novel but had somehow dropped out of medical textbooks and largely out of clinical memory until new circumstances rekindled interest in it.[8] These observations

focused at first on renal complications of three seemingly unrelated occurrences—poisoning by mercuric bichloride (as in the
case that opened this chapter); introduction of a novel class of
drugs, the sulfonamide antimicrobials; and crush injuries to muscle sustained by Londoners during the Battle of Britain (the aerial
bombing of British civilian targets during World War II). Soon,
physicians and surgeons recognized other causes of acute renal
failure, particularly shock. Shock is a response to blood loss, profound dysfunction of the heart, or certain overwhelming infections; its essential features include a marked loss of blood pressure
and failure of the circulation to deliver blood to the body's most
essential organs.

Two unifying themes were selected as cardinal by the clinicians
of the 1940s and 1950s who were formulating the concept of acute
renal failure: sudden loss of renal filtration and thus urine flow,
and potential reversibility. Following the inciting event, urine flow
decreased sharply or stopped altogether, and renally excreted substances (like urea and potassium) built up in the blood—the kidneys effectively shut down operations.[9] Death might occur from
potassium toxicity or uremia—the same uremia that Richard
Bright, William Osler, and Thomas Addis saw, usually in a more
protracted form—but if the patient could hang on, a spontaneous
recovery began with a trickle, or even gush, of urine, characteristi-
cally on day 7 to 14 after the onset of the oliguria. The awareness
that recovery of both kidney and patient could occur, but usually
not before a week had passed, posed a sharp challenge to hospital
physicians dealing with acute renal failure. Some of those who
gained expertise with the disorder argued that physiologically informed management of the quantity and content of diet and fluids ought to be enough to protect the patient during the period of
time without working kidneys. That is, if the intake to the body
could be properly restricted, one could do without the output for
a short time. Others favored use of the new but admittedly hazardous artificial kidney and urged not waiting to use it until the
patient was moribund.[10] A considerable debate ensued between
"dialyzers" and "nondialyzers," though experienced and judicious
authorities such as Merrill understood the role of both types of
treatment.[11]

The several inciting causes of the acute renal failure syndrome illustrate how diseases exist in, and may in fact arise from, a variety of social and medical circumstances delimited in time and place. In the first three decades of the twentieth century, individuals intent on suicide sometimes swallowed mercuric chloride, which was widely available. Occasionally, accidental intake occurred as well, and its use to induce abortion has been horrifically illustrated above. It is not surprising that the "bichloride kidney" as a product of suicide attempts and self-induced abortion became well known during the Great Depression, though it was recognized earlier. The typical symptoms included vomiting, bloody diarrhea, necrotic mouth ulcers, sometimes shock, and anuria (meaning absolutely no urine output) or oliguria. What urine the corroded kidneys managed to produce was often full of blood, casts, and debris but not the marked albuminuria characteristic of Bright's Disease, or glomerulonephritis. Despite the extreme renal injury and dramatic consequences, recovery could occur.[12]

The first important antibacterial drugs, the sulfonamides, appeared in the late 1930s, a discovery of Gerhard Domagk of I.G. Farbenindustrie in Germany. Soon these "sulfa" drugs transformed the treatment of pneumonia, meningitis, and other serious infections. Soon also, a new renal syndrome appeared: sulfonamide-induced acute renal failure. There were actually two adverse reactions. The early sulfa antimicrobials passed from the bloodstream through the glomerular sieves into the tubular fluid, where they sometimes caused trouble by coming out of solution and forming crystals that blocked flow, preventing the formation of adequate amounts of urine. In addition, certain patients unpredictably experienced a hypersensitivity (allergic) reaction to one of these medications. The reaction could cause an inflammatory process in the kidneys in addition to the more familiar allergic skin rash. As case reports gathered in the medical literature, it became clear that both of these forms of sulfa-induced acute renal failure could resolve and the patient recover. (Subsequently, pharmaceutical companies created sulfa-based antibacterial agents with much less propensity to cause either of these toxic effects, several of which remain in regular use today.)[13]

But it was World War II, particularly the bombing of London, that led to the medical reports that most convincingly established the concept of reversible acute renal failure. Eric Bywaters (with Desmond Beall) published the first of his papers on myoglobin-uric renal failure in March of 1941.[14] In this syndrome, crush injury of muscle releases into the blood the substance myoglobin, which especially in the setting of low blood pressure can cause a toxic injury to the kidneys. Bywaters and Beall described the typical story of the London air-raid casualty with this complication:

> The patient has been buried for several hours with pressure on a limb. On admission he looks in good condition except for swelling of the limb, some local anesthesia [numbness of the skin of the injured limb], and whealing. . . . [A] few hours later, despite vasoconstriction, made manifest by pallor, coldness, and sweating, the blood pressure falls. This is restored to pre-shock levels by (often multiple) transfusions of serum, plasma, or, occasionally, blood. . . . Signs of renal damage soon appear, and progress even though the crushed limb be amputated. The urinary output, initially small, owing perhaps to the severity of the shock, diminishes further. The urine contains albumin and many dark brown or black granular casts. These later decrease in number. The patient is alternatively drowsy and anxiously aware of the severity of his illness. Slight generalized oedema, thirst, and incessant vomiting develop, and the blood pressure often remains slightly raised. The blood urea and potassium, raised at an early stage, become progressively higher.

Shock, or extremely low blood pressure, will halt renal filtration and urine formation, since these are driven by circulatory force. But Bywaters and others recognized that something more complex was occurring in the unfortunate victims of the civilian bombings of England. They saw that even when blood pressure was restored by transfusion of plasma or blood, the kidneys remained inactive, at least for a sustained period of time. The four cases reported by Bywaters and Beall were all fatal; but it soon became recognized, as with the bichloride kidney and the sulfonamide renal syndromes, that regeneration of injured kidney cells could occur, and with it, the potential for restoration of well-being to the patient. The recovery would take, usually, at least seven to ten days.

Alert to the syndrome of sudden but reversible renal failure, physicians and surgeons began to detect it in other settings. With battlefield injuries, it was observed that shock alone can incite oliguria or anuria, which would persist even after restoration of blood pressure but might ultimately resolve after several days or weeks. Colonel Balduin Lucké of the U.S. Army Institute of Pathology reported 538 fatal cases in 1946 and provided a label based on his interpretation of the histological pattern he saw: "lower nephron nephrosis." The ungainly name stuck, at least for a time; and a name—especially one that offers the sense of certainty implicit in micropathological diagnosis—helps secure the reality of a "new" disease. A name aids discussion and classification of cases for study, as I have suggested in earlier chapters. Eventually "lower nephron nephrosis" would give way to the term "acute tubular necrosis," which has persisted in use even after it became clear that for certain variations of the syndrome the tubules lacked obvious necrosis (destruction of cells) when renal tissue was examined.[15] Physicians dealing with this entity, mostly nephrologists and their students, always have referred to it using the initials ATN almost as an abstraction, a phrase ("aye-tee-enn") signifying an event more than a pathological appearance. In the early 2000s, the phrase "acute kidney injury" gradually came into use to replace the outdated ATN. Of course, it is shortened to AKI.

The acute renal failure syndrome, or ATN, or "acute kidney injury," highlights the kidney as innocent bystander, a victim of societal malaise, or of medical progress—or of both. Economic depression and the first sustained bombing of civilian populations by aircraft accounted for many of the defining cases, though a welcome new and effective drug provided some others. Even the episodes of acute renal failure caused by the air raids, battlefield wounds, and shock during World War II proclaimed medical advance within the depravity of global warfare: it was only recently perfected methods for resuscitating victims of trauma with transfusions of blood or plasma that allowed them to live long enough to reveal the presence of ATN. Of course, to refer to the kidneys as "innocent bystanders" is something of a conceit: one might say the same thing about other organs, or the whole body for that matter, when considering external injury, exposure to a toxin, or invasion by a microbial pathogen. The liver, for example, might claim innocent bystander status in relation to the viruses that provoke hepatitis, or the excessive drinking of alcohol that brings on cirrhosis. But every substance in the blood passes through the kidneys and becomes concentrated there; and the active cells of the renal tubules require a high rate of oxygen delivery to function and maintain integrity. Thus, the kidneys are particularly vulnerable to injury from toxins, from circulating complexes of unruly antibodies, and from decreased blood flow. Admittedly, they do sometimes seem like feckless and high-strung members of the workforce of organs, a little too willing to sit out a crisis.

Increasingly the offending "nephrotoxins" (toxins to the kidney) have been medications, and some of the episodes of low blood flow to the kidneys have been consequences of surgery and medical procedures. Acute kidney disease since the 1930s and 1940s falls often into the lamented category "iatrogenic"—literally "brought on by the physician," or more broadly, by adverse effects of medicine or surgery. As noted above, often it is a medical success of one sort that, keeping a very sick person alive, allows renal failure to occur as a reaction to some new complication or setback. Acute renal failure can occur as a result not only of shock and "sepsis" (overwhelming infection) but also as a reaction to the dye used for certain radiologic tests, to diagnostic catheterization of the arterial system, and from toxicity of certain antibiotics. As modern medicine established the intensive care unit (ICU) to gather together its most sophisticated tools and efforts for its most ill or injured beneficiaries, ATN chose that place to take up residence. It perniciously persists despite all efforts to avoid it, a by-product of floridly expanding medical capability.[16]

Renal shutdown became an event along the way of the ICU patient's saga, maybe seventh to tenth on the "problem list." A grim witticism in the intensive care setting predicts that when the nephrologist and dialysis nurse are fetched and wheel their apparatus in the direction of a catastrophically ill patient, the minister will be next in line to visit. Indeed, even though renal function can be at least partly replaced by dialysis, survival rates remain poor among very sick hospitalized patients whose course has been impeded by ATN. Even its milder and readily reversible forms, such as that which can on rare occasion follow the use of X-ray contrast, extend the length of the hospital stay and invoke risk.[17] I should point out, however, that many of those severely ill with complicating renal failure do survive only through the support of dialysis, sometimes needing it for many weeks.

The ICU is new, but concern about iatrogenesis is not. In the early nineteenth century, Richard Bright and other British physicians deliberated on the possible role of then ubiquitous mercurial medications (but not the bichloride) in causing dropsy, albuminuria, and renal disease.[18] Bright did not embrace the idea, though he did eventually note that people with renal disease tolerated mercurial drugs poorly, and he prescribed them very little. Well before then, physicians and surgeons (and fearful patients) recognized the risks of paracentesis for dropsy. William Withering showed how to balance the value of foxglove with the plant's toxicity when treating dropsy. Thomas Addis knew that if he pressed the low-protein diet for his renal patients too far, malnutrition could result. "Desperate cases need the most desperate remedies," reads a famous aphorism of Hippocrates, and it has always been so.[19]

The establishment of the ATN syndrome would provide the future nephrologist with that specialist's most frequent and reliable source of consultation in the ICU or hospital room. Certainly the physicians encountered in the previous chapters of this book qualified as owning "special" knowledge of kidney disease—indeed, they created much of it—but the identifiable specialty within medicine devoted to the kidney and its diseases, known as nephrology, did not arise until the 1950s.[20] By "identifiable specialty," I refer to such attributes as membership societies, dedicated periodicals and conferences, and a process for certification. Most essential, of course, is the individual specialist's comprehensive knowledge, theoretical and practical. Applying specialist knowledge, the renal physician could help distinguish ATN from extrarenal failure (renal dysfunction from inadequate blood flow to kidneys, later called prerenal azotemia) or other disorders that might also present with oliguria and uremia. These included certain forms of acute glomerulonephritis, formerly called acute

Bright's Disease, and a myriad of rare and weirdly named diseases that would win their place in textbook lists.[21]

From the 1960s on, interpretation of urinary chemical measurements enhanced the traditional inspection of urine sediment in sorting out what has gone wrong with the kidneys, and both formed part of the nephrologist's consultation for "oliguria and rising creatinine." The specialist's contribution of course extended beyond diagnosis, and by the late 1940s physicians with particular interest in disorders of the kidney could supervise management of diet and fluids, or even, in some few hospitals, set up the artificial kidney. Indeed, many specialties have in good part depended upon a captured technical element for their success—the electrocardiograph and echocardiogram of the cardiologist, the various 'scopes of the otolaryngologist or gastroenterologist.

THE SPREAD OF DIALYSIS FOR ACUTE RENAL FAILURE

Overcoming considerable uncertainty about its value, hemodialysis became a routine part of caring for acute renal failure during the late 1940s and 1950s. Convinced of the device's worth, internist George Thorn (1906–2004) of Boston's Peter Bent Brigham Hospital and Harvard Medical School stimulated the construction of an improved stainless steel version of the Kolff rotating-drum artificial kidney by a mechanically minded surgical colleague, Carl Walter (1905–1992), and an engineer-machinist named Edward Olson. Thorn assigned a young physician trainee in his department, the aforementioned John P. Merrill, to direct application of dialysis at "the Brigham." There, it won markers of an accepted technology: its own place, attendants, and replication. The hospital assigned space for a dialysis "unit," in which two persons could be treated. Research nurse Barbara Coleman Wysocki found herself the first dialysis nurse and technician in the United States. As with another increasingly technological clinical space, the operating room, regular use of the artificial kidney came to require a multidisciplinary clinical "team," one of many that would arise in medicine. By the end of the twentieth century, "teamwork" and "teaching teamwork" reached the top of the favorite-phrase list within the rhetoric of American medical education.

The Brigham-Kolff dialyzer proved sufficiently successful that it was manufactured and sold during the 1950s to hospitals in North and South America and Europe. In Washington, D.C., it was used at the hospital of Georgetown University and at the Walter Reed Army Research Institute. Physicians working at these centers, some of whom had done training with the nascent dialysis center in Boston, brought about the use of the dialyzer at an evacuation hospital near Pusan during the Korean War. It is generally held that its ability to prevent death from hyperkalemia (retention of potassium, causing malfunction of the heart) among injured soldiers with acute renal failure powerfully advanced the reputation of hemodialysis as an effective and practicable modality. In France, dialysis for acute renal failure began in Paris under Maurice Dérot and Marcel Legrain at the Hotel Dieu in 1949, and later under Jean Hamburger and Gabriel Richet at Hôpital Necker.

During the 1950s, physicians interested in, and unafraid of, the artificial kidney began to form an informal network, particularly through Boston-Paris connections.[22] By 1960, although some Kolff-Brigham dialyzers that had been ambitiously purchased gathered dust in the closets of small hospitals, many major centers routinely carried out dialysis for cases of presumed reversible acute renal failure. Soon they retired their Kolff-Brigham behemoths in favor of the more convenient machine manufactured by Travenol Laboratories of Illinois (later acquired by other companies). The Travenol system offered presterilized and—emblematically modern and American—disposable filters and blood lines. Authors of textbooks included dialysis as part of standard care for certain individuals with acute renal failure. Certainly not all physicians and surgeons acquired familiarity with its deployment, but its use became a routine part of training programs within the new specialty centered on kidney diseases now known as nephrology.[23]

RENAL BIOPSY

Also by the late 1940s, and more so into the 1950s and 1960s, some early renal specialists could utilize another device—the biopsy needle. In puzzling or uncertain cases of acute renal failure, perhaps when recovery failed to occur within the expected interval, a specially designed "cutting needle" could be quickly probed into the kidney through the overlying skin and body wall (numbed with a local anesthetic agent). The tiny sliver of renal tissue so obtained is then prepared for inspection under the microscope. For the first time, the pathological appearance of the diseased kidney could be determined in the living patient; and pathology (first whole-kidney, then microscopic) had been the foundation for classifying and making sense of renal disease since the work of Richard Bright. Percutaneous biopsy of the kidney, to use its proper name, was a European invention based on similar methods already applied to the liver and certain tumors. In one of their early papers first describing the technique and its results, Danish physicians Poul Iversen and Claus Brun wrote:

> The conditions in which the renal biopsy technics [*sic*] will presumably be of greatest value are those mild renal disorders which only rarely come to autopsy and also the initial stages of the severe, acute renal disorders. A group of diseases especially useful to examine in greater detail by means of biopsy is that of the acute anurias occurring after shock, utero-placental damage, poisoning with sulfonamides or corrosive sublimate, enteritis, and from many other causes. At present, it is common usage to classify all these conditions under the term "lower nephron nephrosis," but it is doubtful whether such generalization is permissible, and a closer investigation of the histological changes in milder, non-fatal cases of this nature is much needed.[24]

Although acute renal failure remained a subject for biopsy, its use quickly broadened on both sides of the Atlantic. Alvin E. Parrish of George Washington University and the Veterans Administration Hospital in Washington, D.C., was among the first Americans to report a large series of persons evaluated with renal biopsy, most of whose slides showed glomerulonephritis or nephrosclerosis.[25] A more important figure in advancing renal biopsy was Robert M. Kark (1911–2002), a physician born in South Africa who did some of his medical training at Guy's Hospital, where Bright had worked. Another émigré attracted to the United States by postwar opportunities within medical science, Kark spent most of his career in Chicago. He is credited with establishing the clinical and investigational worth (and, no small thing, safety) of renal biopsy, at least in the United States. With clinical colleagues and collaborating pathologists, Kark beginning in the 1950s published a sequence of major research papers clarifying and redefining glomerular disease, especially nephrotic syndrome. This group was joined by others, as the procedure enjoyed technical refinements and proved (in Kark's words) "generally applicable to the sick."[26]

The early nephrologists doing biopsies and their pathologist collaborators had to arrive at new visual standards, since their experience with renal histology until the 1950s rested on tissue obtained from autopsies. Such material mostly represented the end stage of disease and was subject to artifacts occurring after death. Percutaneous biopsy of the living, on the other hand, as Iversen and Brun asserted, could obtain samples (albeit tiny ones) from individuals with early disease, and free of postmortem changes. Biopsy then could establish a diagnosis and help select therapy for a patient when it might matter most—before progression to a terminal phase of disease. Although some criticized the procedure as dangerous, typically for this period physicians both in Europe and North America assumed great freedom and autonomy as they biopsied, looked, interpreted, and published. The early application of the artificial kidney displayed the same sense of adventure and license: "informed consent" and "liability" were not subjects of anxious deliberation in that period. By the mid- to late 1960s, renal biopsy was nearly a matter of routine, an expected skill of the nephrologist. In the 1970s, electron microscopy with its spectacularly high magnification and clarity added to the information that could be obtained from the minute specimen: this was probably the first regular use of electron microscopy for clinical diagnosis. It hardly needs be pointed out that renal biopsy, eventually made safer by the use of ultrasound or CT scans to guide the needle, represented a thoroughly high-technology way to look at the sick kidney.

Paradoxically, by the 1960s it came to be used not so much for exploring the "new" disease of the ICU called acute renal failure but rather for the original problem—proteinuric kidney disease, Bright's Disease. That is, biopsy found its greatest value in establishing a precise pathological diagnosis in cases of what by the time of its invention had come to be known as nephrotic

syndrome—severe proteinuria (albuminuria) with consequent
edema, caused by some disease process attacking mainly the renal
sieves, the glomeruli. And, by discovering—or, in a way, creating—an impossibly complex number of patterns of glomerular
structural abnormalities, renal biopsy rejuvenated the study of
what once had been Bright's Disease. But biopsy also completed
the destruction of "Bright's Disease" as a name and as a sickness
that held meaning for both patients and doctors. The new proteinuric disorders largely defined by renal biopsy and the electron
microscopy include: membranous nephropathy; minimal change
disease; membranoproliferative glomerulonephritis (types 1 and
2); IgA nephropathy; focal segmental glomerulosclerosis, or FSGS
(comprising five subtypes, such as the "tip variant" and the "collapsing variant").[27] Some of these admittedly ridiculous-sounding
entities do have associations and distinctions beyond the microscope slide. Minimal change disease commonly causes nephrotic
syndrome in children and responds well to treatment. Membranoproliferative glomerulonephritis in the 1990s was linked to infection with hepatitis virus of the C type. FSGS, which often causes
extreme proteinuria and hypertension, occurs for some unknown
reason disproportionately among persons of color, while IgA nephropathy rarely does.

It is hard to know what to say historically about these diseases
of the kidney, or more precisely, of the glomerulus of the kidney.
Certainly the names represent a continuation of the dominant
nineteenth-century way of conducting medicine and medical science, namely, nosology, or disease classification based upon pathological appearance. "Focal segmental glomerulosclerosis, collapsing variant," one might argue, merely carries that approach to a
reductionist extreme and is not different in kind from the "granular kidney" of Bright or "nephrosclerosis" of Volhard and Fahr, or
examples from other earlier categorization schemes not discussed
in this book. On the horizon as I write this are classifications based
on alterations in the numerous structural proteins constituting the
filtration membranes of the glomerulus or based on their genes.
But even if practitioners from the 1850s to the 1940s knew something of the underlying pathological fine print of their day (and
only some would), they could still rely on "Bright's Disease" when

talking with the patient and family; and as we have seen, physician and patient together could share some understanding—and some fear—of its meaning.

Now, Bright's Disease is gone, and it proves perplexing to hold a conversation announcing "membranous nephropathy" or "minimal change disease" to a patient or family. Whereas these increasingly arcane and specific names may foster precision in communications among nephrologists and pathologists, they can only bewilder patients and even general physicians. The situation is made worse by the lack of any available sort of story of cause and effect. For the majority of these biopsy-diagnosed successors to Bright's Disease, the cause is unknown, at least in the sense sought by patient and doctor: "No, as far as we know, it just came of itself—no relation to the cough you had last month, the medication you took last year, drinking too much or too little water, or in fact anything you did or did not do." It should not surprise that too much alcohol, or exposure to cold and wet, survived and served so long as the causes of dropsy, then of Bright's Disease. Those causal connections that made some sense of illness may now be looked upon as wrong. But little satisfaction derives from our (nephrologists') current willing awareness of ignorance: we refer to these disorders as idiopathic, which means something like "it's its own cause."

Understanding the distinctions between the glomerular disorders, recognizing their appearances under the microscope, and keeping up on the clinical trials that inform their treatment all represent the esoteric knowledge of the specialist, the nephrologist (who may also have carried out the biopsy procedure itself). Indeed, the modern medical specialist usually claims three sorts of expertise: practical knowledge (such as rules of diagnosis and treatment); usually some body of abstract theoretical knowledge that nonspecialists cannot master and don't care about; and, often, some technique, as suggested earlier also in relation to dialysis. I have endeavored to make this book a story of kidney disease and persons suffering with it, and not an account of a medical specialty. But another aphorism of Hippocrates declared that the patient, the disease, and the physician constitute a triad.[28] Whereas general physicians (family doctors and general internists) comfortably treat the common diseases of the heart and gastrointestinal tract, the two hallmarks of a serious kidney malady—proteinuria, rising blood creatinine—very often lead to a referral to the nephrologist. The complexity and obtuseness of the proteinuric diseases, as spun out by biopsy, account for this, as does the apprehension that at some point dialysis might be required. By approximately the 1960s, kidney trouble was shifting from the general world of diseases and doctors to the rarified domain of specialists.

Finally, these numerous proteinuric disorders enjoy the bureaucratic sanctioning of ICD codes (International Classification of Diseases), a necessity within the impenetrable billing apparatus of American medicine. They occupy sections 581 and 582, which are, not surprisingly, redundant and confused. Still, as little meaning as "membranoproliferative glomerulonephritis" may have for someone afflicted with it, or the patient's family doctor, at least the name can help get the bills paid.

Renal biopsy during the 1960s and 1970s also added to knowledge of another glomerular and proteinuric renal disease mainly recognized in the 1930s but considered rare—diabetic nephropathy. Though the so-called primary or idiopathic glomerular disorders, discussed above, can sometimes eventually destroy kidney function and lead to uremia, into the 1970s and beyond it would be diabetic kidney disease that became epidemic, the new Bright's Disease of its day. High blood pressure (hypertension) also seemed everywhere, another disease of modern industrial life, and it, too, turned out to be a frequent source of renal damage. Unhappily, diabetes and hypertension are frequent companions. Meanwhile, the artificial kidney underwent enormous refinement and saw expansion of its arena, especially once physicians and surgeons had contrived methods for repeating treatments indefinitely to keep alive persons with burnt-out kidneys incapable of recovery. The less curable of the ICD 581 and 582 diseases, diabetic nephropathy and hypertensive nephrosclerosis, met the new capabilities of the artificial kidney in the *chronic dialysis unit,* an invention in some ways more strange and remarkable than the artificial kidney itself.

—◦◦◦—

A Later Perspective

The cause of acute renal failure in the ICU of the early twenty-first century is often termed "multifactorial," a consequence of more than one factor in very ill people, usually a mixture of serious infection, hypotension, and sometimes toxic effects of necessary drugs. Nephrologists assisting in the care of such persons now utilize, and argue the merits of, a number of variant dialysis methods. Much debate centers on how early to start dialytic treatment in a person with acute renal failure and how often to carry out treatments. Dialysis itself and the blood lines needed to implement it add their own risk. The focus has been on reducing these while achieving adequate control of uremia and fluid retention in an effort to improve the chances of survival for the severely ill.

Nephrology in the United States and Great Britain arose as a specialty centered, of course, on diseases of the kidney and their treatments. Particularly within medical schools and their hospitals in the United States, a strong interest in exploring the normal physiology of the kidney shaped the specialty, as did a similar fascination with the so-called acid-base and electrolyte (sodium and potassium) disorders. The kidneys play a dominant role in acid-base and electrolyte physiology. Dialysis and renal biopsy remain the primary procedures associated with the nephrologist, who now devotes much of his or her working hours to the care of people on chronic dialysis (chapter 6). The specialty's organizations include the International Society of Nephrology and the American Society of Nephrology. Both publish respected scientific and clinical journals.

Renal biopsy is still called upon occasionally in perplexing cases of acute renal failure. It remains in daily use primarily for the diagnosis of glomerular diseases such as those mentioned earlier—for example, membranous nephropathy, minimal change disease, FSGS, and IgA nephropathy. The ability of biopsy to designate "new" renal diseases, or new subtypes of old ones, seems boundless. Even if the cause of these glomerular diseases remains unknown in most cases, the differentiation can claim some value. The prognosis varies, and that is often a useful piece of information to know, something patients often wish to hear. Perhaps more importantly, there is treatment that can be tried for most of these entities, mainly cortisone-type steroids and a variety of other drugs that work by suppressing certain elements of the immune system, such as cyclo-phosphamide, azathioprine, or the newer mycophenolate mofetil. Most of the drugs used were devised first for use in treating can-cer or preventing rejection of a transplanted organ. Some overac-tivity or other malfunction of the body's immune systems seems to be at play in at least many of the glomerular "nephropathies." What works for minimal change disease, however, generally fails for membranous nephropathy, which is considered responsive to something different, and so on. So, it is important to know the exact, "biopsy-proved" diagnosis. The selected treatments are by no means "magic bullets," certain and specific to the particular spe-cies of disorder. In fact, they fall more into the category of roughly aimed shotguns, only sometimes effective, always dangerous. The modern controlled clinical trial has been increasingly called upon to establish the true effectiveness of these drugs in the various types of glomerular disorders. Unfortunately, results of one trial do not always confirm the findings of the previous ones, and considerable uncertainty remains.

Biopsy is also used to identify the source of poor functioning in transplanted kidneys. That is, examination of the specimen enables the nephrologist and surgeon to decide if the problem is rejection of the kidney by the body's immune system, a drug toxicity, or some other disturbance. Some transplant programs carry out biop-sies on a planned schedule or "protocol" to detect difficulties at an early stage, or as part of research.

Increasingly, and throughout the Western world, the leading single cause of glomerular disease (and of chronic, irreversible renal failure) is diabetes. Both the so-called type 1 (formerly "juvenile") and the far more common type 2 (adult-onset) can, over long pe-riods of time, injure the kidney. Tighter control of the blood sugar can reduce the risk of renal complications, as does normalization of concurrent high blood pressure. Several classes of medication that reduce activity of a prohypertensive substance called angiotensin seem to be especially beneficial in persons with diabetes. As noted in chapter 4, some parasitic infections lead to a glomerular reac-tion, making them the dominant source of proteinuria and failing kidneys in some parts of the world, particularly Africa.

CHAPTER SIX

Inventing
Chronic Dialysis

Like chapter 1, this chapter begins with an illustration of a person in a chair. This man has not taken to a chair in his home, but rather sits in a strange medical space newly created in the second half of the twentieth century—the chronic dialysis unit, or dialysis clinic. He is one of thirty people occupying one of thirty chairs in this particular dialysis unit in Philadelphia, one of about 300,000 such patients in the United States (in the early twenty-first century), about one million in the world.[1] Some years ago, after a long period of decline, his kidneys reached the point of almost no activity at all, a circumstance at one time, of course, incompatible with life. But he reports to this chair three times a week for four hours at a time to receive treatments from the most modern, computerized version of the artificial kidney—which is the apparatus to his left, topped by its digital display. The treatment is referred to as chronic dialysis or maintenance dialysis. The hemodialysis machine, aided by certain medications and—as with past patients with Bright's Disease, dietary restrictions—keeps the gentleman alive and feeling tolerably well. The treatment leaves him free of dropsy and prevents the violent symptoms of uremia—the vomiting, pains, and seizures that afflicted some patients of Richard Bright, James Tyson, and Thomas Addis.

He lacks the stamina he once had when he worked as a warehouse foreman, but like many of his copatients in the other chairs,

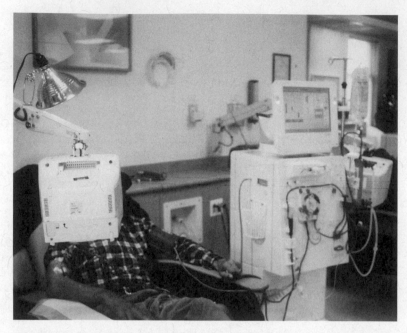

A patient receiving a hemodialysis treatment in a chronic dialysis unit in Philadelphia with which the author has been associated. Photograph by the author. Reproduced with permission of
the patient.

few of whom are able to hold jobs, his age alone would allow retirement. For younger Americans in his circumstances, it is fortu-
nate that the U.S. federal government in 1972 declared complete
failure of the kidneys a form of "disability," making its treatment
with thrice-weekly dialysis eligible for coverage under Medicare
regardless of age. This decision also created something like another new name for Bright's Disease: the man in the photograph
and those like him have "end-stage renal disease," or ESRD, a
nosologic category based on entitlement, not pathology. This African-American man lost his kidney function over a long period of
time from hypertension (high blood pressure); it would have occurred sooner had he not shown admirable diligence in taking his
three or four different blood pressure medications and never missing an appointment with his physician (the author). For reasons
still not fully clear, American blacks suffer ESRD at a rate three

to four times that of white persons and are particularly vulnerable to renal injury from hypertension (this is not unique to American persons of color). African Americans fill dialysis chairs throughout the inner cities of the United States.

Let us reconsider the chair. The dropsical patient of old resorted to the chair in misery—ill and weak, she could not enjoy even the small comfort of the sickbed because lying down made the fluid choke off breath. For the dialysis patient, in contrast, the chair came to represent the aspiration to health. In the infancy of repeated dialysis for irreversible kidney failure, patients received their treatments in hospital *beds,* wearing hospital garb, even when no longer inpatients. Soon, it seemed obviously more practical to allow patients coming in to the dialysis unit for treatments to remain in normal clothing, and to receive their treatments in a chair. They underwent a sort of optimistic redefinition, from *patients* in gowns and beds, to *persons* with a manageable condition that merely required a visit to a special treatment center for a few hours several times per week. One man, a writer, receiving dialysis in the 1970s described what he saw at his first visit to a New York City dialysis center this way: "The patients were in street clothes, sitting in reclining lounge chairs, reading, watching TV sets, chatting with one another, even taking tiny sips of coffee or tea from plastic cups, or sucking chips of ice."[2] Dialysis units indeed use recliners, a piece of affordable luxury prevalent in American dens and family rooms.

But the choice signifies something else within the dialysis center—in fact, it is still a place of sickness, and sometimes, no matter how well dressed he or she may be, a patient's blood pressure drops to nothing as the machine draws off over a few hours fluid that was ingested over two days. Then, down go the back of the chair and the patient's head (like when someone feels faint) as the nursing staff react almost by instinct to correct the loss of equilibrium. The attendant will rapidly infuse some saline (in the plastic bag seen hanging from a pole) to raise the blood pressure. Chronic dialysis cannot be considered, even almost fifty years since its beginnings, an entirely carefree way to pass time.

In our photograph, the small suspended television hides the subject's face. I posed it this way purposely, to maintain his privacy.

(I am writing this book in the early years of HIPAA, the U.S. government's Health Insurance Portability and Accountability Act, which has fostered an almost hysterical frenzy for confidentiality and the signing of forms.) He would not have objected to showing his identity had I asked (I have known the man for over twenty years), and nothing about being a chronic dialysis patient need cause shame. Indeed, such a life can demand courage, patience, resolve, tolerance, and easily a half-dozen other virtues. Many individuals do watch TV as their hours of treatment drag by.

It is not entirely coincidental that the artificial kidney and the television set are nearly contemporaneous technologies: they have grown up together since the late 1940s in a world continuously abloom with unexpected machines and devices. They have also grown smaller together, the effect of engineering advances, especially in solid-state electronics. The hours weigh heavily on dialysis recipients, and television excels at sponging up time. Unfortunately, many patients during the treatments experience muscle cramps, the hypotensive episodes mentioned above, occasional need to reposition the needles that convey blood to and from the "access," and other discomforts and distractions. Depending upon the location of the "access to circulation," a surgically altered vein or implanted artificial blood vessel, one arm might need to be kept still. The gentleman in the photograph has an access in his right arm, and one can trace the path of the blood lines from the machine to that arm. A cuff for monitoring blood pressure claims his left arm. Furthermore, in a busy unit containing twenty or thirty machines and patients, looked after by a crowd of nurses and technicians, some alarm or monitor is always beeping against a background of professional chatter and episodic cajoling or scolding. Thus, carrying out some more active occupation, which patients might otherwise choose, even reading, can prove difficult. Of course, many now use headphones or earbuds with personal music devices to dwell in some more agreeable private place. And, as noted above, some who are medically stable do manage to read, study, finish paperwork.

I referred above to the blood lines, the flexible plastic tubes that connect the dialysis filter (the cylindrical structure in the clamp at the far right of the image) to the recipient's bloodstream by way of the hollow needles inserted into one or another form of the access to circulation, that is, a fistula or graft. Between human and machine, we view an intimate connection: not just *any* body fluid, or ancient humor, but blood itself circulates continuously, for hours at a time, from one to the other. The relationship lacks balance, however, for the patient's life depends upon the machine. It is not surprising that for some such persons, the machine becomes a friend, even a part of the family for those who learn to operate it and perform their treatments at home. One grateful patient in Georgia came to see the machine as "a friend—a life-long friend, at that," while another's family (doing dialysis at home) named their artificial kidney apparatus "Fred."[3] Many others are unable to reach such acceptance. "I don't want to be buddy-buddy with the machine," said one, angrily, when dialysis at home was suggested. "It's a machine—if it does its job, I'll do mine."[4] (The patient's "job" will receive a description in chapter 7.) Another said: "The machine becomes a part of you. But it never becomes a friend. You have no choice unless you want to push up daisies. And I don't—yet."[5]

THE DEVELOPMENT OF CHRONIC DIALYSIS

It is not entirely clear what sort of patients troubled the minds of the medical tinkerers of the 1940s (and even before) who built the first, clumsy artificial kidney machines in Europe and North America. As we saw in chapter 5, the recognition of the reversible acute renal failure syndrome certainly justified the efforts. It powerfully appealed to clinical logic: acutely injured kidneys often will get better after a nearly predictable period of nonfunction; but patients may feel wretchedly ill and even die during the phase of complete shutdown; the artificial kidney used once or a few times can reduce the symptoms, correct the chemical derangements, and put off death; once renal regeneration occurred, it need visit that patient no more. The dialysis machine appears as a specific treatment prescribed for a limited time, facilitating if not precisely creating a cure. But pioneers of hemodialysis in the 1950s like Nils Alwall, Willem J. Kolff, and John P. Merrill all occasionally offered treatment with the artificial kidney to people with known chronic, irreversible disease. They did so when they believed that some transient stress, such as infection, dehydration, or surgery, had caused a symptomatic but *reversible* decompensation in a person with chronic disease not yet in its terminal phase. Such an individual once past the destabilizing event might regain enough renal function to return to a viable, even if marginal, condition.

Kolff and others also believed that dialytic treatment of symptomatic uremia could sometimes improve appetite and lessen uremic nausea enough for the sufferer to begin eating a therapeutic diet, low in protein and sodium, that would itself control symptoms. In fact, all the early dialysis physicians occasionally saw chronic patients regain for a period of months a sense of well-being through episodic use of the artificial kidney. The ethical dangers in this attempt were expressed by the early nephrology specialist John Merrill in 1955 with his customary humanity and lucid language: "The ability to restore a convulsing, comatose patient with irreversible chronic renal failure to a state of well-being and good appetite is an accomplishment which must not be unwisely utilized. False hopes engendered in the minds of patient and the family by this phenomenon are all the more tragic when the signs and symptoms begin to recur within a matter of days. . . . The decision to employ dialysis in chronic renal failure is one not lightly to be arrived at, and requires a full understanding of the many problems, both physiologic and sociologic."[6]

The extension of hemodialysis to *long-term replacement of renal function* for chronic cases began in the United States with the work of Belding Scribner (1921–2003).[7] Scribner first took interest in renal disease when he was a medical student in Thomas Addis's elective course at Stanford University School of Medicine in the 1940s. Following his postgraduate training in internal medicine, Scribner went to Seattle to join the staff of that city's Veterans Administration Hospital and the faculty of the University of Washington School of Medicine. During the 1950s he carried out research dealing with bedside methods of chemical analysis (e.g., for bicarbonate, urea) and disorders of potassium balance. While doing some additional training at the Mayo Clinic in Rochester, Minnesota, Scribner had heard a presentation on dialysis by John Merrill, who was visiting from Boston. Scribner has recounted his career in terms of particular patients' plights, as did dialysis inventor Willem Kolff before him. In 1960 a man named Joe Saunders came to the University of Washington Hospital with a diagnosis of acute renal failure.

> When he entered the hospital, he was in coma, and his heart failure was so bad that foam was oozing out of his lungs and mouth. Yet one week [after dialysis began] Joe was up and about, feeling amazingly well as a result of several treatments on the artificial kidney . . . and yet despite this amazing result all was not right. Mr. Saunders had not passed any urine in a week, a fact that made the original diagnosis suspect. A biopsy of his kidney revealed the tragic answer. The original diagnosis was wrong. Mr. Saunders had a disease which had totally and irreversibly destroyed his kidneys. They would never function again.
>
> What to do? . . . We did the only thing we could do. We had an agonizing conversation with Mrs. Saunders and told her to take her husband back home to Spokane where he would die.
>
> Then one morning about 4:00 a.m. I woke up and groped for a piece of paper and pencil to jot down the basic idea of the shunted cannulas which would make it possible to treat people like Joe Saunders again and again with the artificial kidney without destroying two blood vessels each time.[8]

As reported by Scribner in his initial 1960 publications about the device, Nils Alwall had attempted to create a mechanical "shunt" for dialysis in 1949 as part of his experimental work using rabbits, so the concept was not new.[9] The fundamental idea was this: a cannula, or small flexible tube, is sewn into an artery, and another into a vein at the wrist. These allow connection to the artificial kidney during treatments: arterial blood goes out and through the filter, with return into the vein. The two cannulae are connected through a shunt when dialysis is not being done. Except when dialysis is underway, the recipient could simply wrap the external shunt in some gauze and go about his or her business. The rapid, shunted flow of blood from artery to vein would prevent clotting or occlusion of the tubes between uses. Scribner and engineer Wayne Quinton succeeded by choosing suitable materials and contour to oppose both bleeding and clotting.

Scribner's team placed a working shunt in their first selected patient with chronic disease, a man named Clyde Shields, on March 9, 1960, within a few months of initiating its development. Shields was able to undergo intermittent dialytic treatment without rapid consumption of his blood vessels and would remain alive, but dependent on the artificial kidney, for ten years. By May of 1960, Scribner and his nurses kept four patients in Seattle alive, if not always robustly well, using hemodialysis and the Quinton-Scribner shunt. The days of exuberant medical freedom and adventure, exemplified in nephrology by the artificial kidney and needle biopsy, were, however, approaching an end, at least for Scribner: the University of Washington Hospital foresaw the soaring cost of the innovation and ordered him to accept no more candidates for chronic hemodialysis.[10] The shunt, along with improved filters and other apparatus, provided the technical capability for extending hemodialysis to persons with irreversibly failed kidneys, but a social and economic mechanism had to be found.

Scribner conceived of a community dialysis center to which patients would come several times each week for treatments, though he later encouraged dialysis at home once that seemed safe and feasible. To fund the novel idea of a community dialysis unit, Scribner, like many American predecessors in renal research, called upon foundation philanthropy. He applied to the John A. Hartford Foundation, a product of the A&P grocery store company, which in the 1950s had supported renal dialysis and transplantation in Boston. The Hartford Foundation for a time served as the particular patron of the artificial kidney. It aided Scribner's program until 1967.[11]

The Seattle Artificial Kidney Center (SAKC), the first dialysis unit for outpatients, opened in January of 1962 in Seattle's Swedish Hospital. Chronic dialysis units dwelled at first within hospitals as a kind of transitional strategy that provided for backup in case of emergencies. Later, most such units would be freestanding, occupying rented or owned space in urban downtowns and neighborhoods, or in the suburbs. Early centers usually could carry out two to four dialysis treatments simultaneously, but eventually this number rose to twenty or more. Engineer Albert Babb working with Scribner's team devised a system to continuously produce the necessary dialysate solution and send it to each of the multiple machines in use. The large chronic outpatient dialysis unit became something entirely new in medicine and a novel application of assembly-line methods. Recipients typically appear three times each week (Mondays, Wednesdays, and Fridays or Tuesdays, Thursdays, and Saturdays). They occupy a chair while connected to a dialysis machine for three to five hours, have their blood and bodies cleared of uremic toxins and excess fluid, and—when all proceeds well—go home. The "unit" (in a different sense) of the earliest days of dialysis—single severely sick patient, doctor, nurse, and mechanic—gave way to *shifts* of patients (up to three shifts per day) and of staff; *batching* of dialysate; and prodigious consumption of disposable dialysis filters, needles, and tubing. Automation controlled the distribution of the dialysate solutions and guided the blood flows and pressure adjustments for each person and machine, as the technology advanced from the 1960s onward.

Ironically, Belding Scribner himself increasingly favored the alternative plan of training recipients and family members to carry out dialysis at home, which allowed for a more flexible schedule, greater patient autonomy, and reduced risk of certain infections. Scribner combined a fondness for things mechanical (he loved flying radio-controlled model airplanes) with an ability to create and guide organizational structures, the optimal mixture to establish chronic dialysis as a reality. He would later in his life decry for-profit dialysis.[12]

GROWTH AND SUPPORT OF CHRONIC DIALYSIS IN THE UNITED STATES

The experience in Seattle encouraged other renal physicians in the United States to learn the placement and care of shunts and to begin using dialysis to treat chronic kidney disease. These included George Schreiner in Washington, Willem Kolff in Cleveland, John Merrill in Boston, and a few others already skilled in short-term dialysis. Other specialists in kidney diseases in the United States, especially those more concerned with normal and disordered renal physiology, expressed skepticism: they believed that chronic dialysis should not spread unchecked without a more scientific assessment.[13] And most of those trying to replicate Scribner's success found that at least for some years, they could not—complications, frustration, and unexpected deaths filled the newly founded units.

Still, no one could deny that many people with terminal kidney failure were being kept alive, if not entirely well, by the artificial kidney. In 1963 the U.S. government became active in the expansion of maintenance dialysis care when the Veterans Administration began its construction of thirty dialysis units within its hospital system. In 1965 the U.S. Public Health Service created its Kidney Disease Control Program, which awarded funds for development of fourteen "demonstration" chronic dialysis units based at hospitals in major cities.[14] Many units sprang up without federal backing, and a few states created limited programs to support maintenance dialysis. A compilation of "kidney disease services, facilities and programs in the United States" published in May of 1969, but probably assembled in 1968, showed that only eight states lacked any maintenance dialysis services, and at least nine states claimed ten or more units. By 1970, maintenance dialysis kept alive over 2,500 Americans and over 3,000 Europeans, as well as unknown numbers in Japan and possibly a few other countries.[15] By this time, a major technical improvement in "access to the circulation"—the arteriovenous fistula described by Michael Brescia, James Cimino, and Keith Appel of New York City—began to replace the shunt.[16] The shunt certainly had done the job and made chronic dialysis possible, but its vulnerability to clotting and infection harried the days and nights of patients and staff.

In the earliest years of chronic dialysis, the number of people who might benefit from the procedure exceeded its availability. In fact, the SAKC became the locus for one of the signal case studies in twentieth-century bioethics. Given the limited capacity and uncertainty about how patients of various sorts would respond, Scribner and colleagues drew up seemingly reasonable medical criteria. Persons accepted for maintenance dialysis would have to be age forty-five or younger and free of major systemic diseases— that is, they would have isolated kidney disease, which would usually have been from some form of chronic glomerulonephritis (i.e., "Bright's Disease" were that term still used). But the medical criteria did not sufficiently bring the number of potential recipients in balance with the number of available dialysis "slots."

The Seattle physicians thus came up with the idea that a panel of laypersons in the community, joined by physicians, could create and implement other sorts of criteria to determine who, among those deemed medically appropriate, would receive the life-extending therapy. Named the Admissions and Policy Committee, it and the artificial kidney gained widespread recognition through an article in *Life* magazine of November 1972 by journalist Shana Alexander titled "They Decide Who Lives, Who Dies: Medical Miracle Puts Moral Burden on a Small Committee."[17] The lay committee members weighed attributes that might, or might not, place a potential recipient of dialysis in the social sphere they knew and valued. They gave precedence mainly to those with families, especially working heads of households, and also considered whether a candidate contributed to the community and went to church. When viewed as excessively favoring middle-class ways of being, the process attracted much criticism.[18]

It has sometimes been assumed that all of the early chronic dialysis units appointed similar lay admissions committees, but in fact few did. More often, physicians and staff of the unit formed an approval committee that emphasized mainly prognosis and other medical criteria (freedom from diseases other than kidney failure, likelihood of being able to comply with the treatment program). These committees did to a lesser extent consider other factors, such as "intelligence in relation to understanding treatment," family support, and absence of criminal background.

Whatever the criteria may have been, no doubt many persons with irreversible kidney disease in the 1960s in the United States and elsewhere did not receive maintenance dialysis and died, though the actual numbers are unknown. One estimate, based on uncertain projections from death certificates and several assumptions, placed the number of persons who might have been eligible for dialysis in the United States in 1964 at approximately 6,400, a time when only several hundred obtained such treatment.[19] I can remember clearly from my years as a medical student and resident physician in the late 1960s and first few years of the 1970s that some practitioners sending patients to a medical school hospital had never heard of chronic hemodialysis. Elderly patients with renal failure, and some with multiple complications of diabetes, received only a restricted diet, the newly available "loop" diuretics to force the small remaining amount of working kidney to squeeze out a bit more salt and water, and other measures aimed at relieving symptoms. Still, it is clear that by 1970 a considerable number of young (or at least not very old), otherwise healthy Americans with terminal kidney disease, living in urban areas, did find their way to dialysis. They constituted the 2,500 patients cited above.

The considerable expenses of the treatment were met by a few state programs, the Veterans Administration for veterans, the U.S. Public Health Service for its "demonstration" units, occasionally by private insurance, or through family support and community fund-raising. No doubt, however, many people needing dialysis, some unable to work, still confronted unceasing financial stress that added to their burden of disease.[20] In the context of American society in the 1960s, one has to suspect that fewer otherwise appropriate poor persons with kidney failure found a chair at a chronic unit than those more affluent. Yet, as early as 1973—the first year of the Medicare program to pay for dialysis (discussed below)—actual counts of patients already showed that the proportion of black Americans receiving the treatment was two to three times higher than that for whites.[21]

Maintenance dialysis in the United States during the 1960s presented an entirely novel dilemma in health care that became understood with this formulation: a modern, proven medical "miracle" in the form of a machine can save lives otherwise prematurely lost; but supplying and staffing this particular miracle make it extraordinarily expensive, and not all Americans can afford it; thus Americans, citizens of the world's richest country, are suffering "needless deaths" for want of funds to obtain the treatment.[22] A remarkable resolution of the dilemma occurred on October 30, 1972, when President Richard M. Nixon signed into law P.L. 92-603, a set of Social Security amendments, section 2991 of which effectively committed the federal Medicare program to pay for chronic dialytic care and renal transplantation. This unique legislation resulted from a complex political process that has been recounted by Richard Rettig, Reneé Fox and Judith Swazey, and others and will be retold here only briefly.[23] Federal payment for care of persons with one particular disease had no precedent, but the lawmaking proceeded within a context. Several influential senators and representatives favored extending Medicare coverage beyond those over sixty-five to the disabled of any age. Some sympathy also existed for coverage of "catastrophic" disease.

All who have studied the genesis of the chronic kidney disease amendment have stressed the importance of "identified lives"— real persons whom lawmakers could see (and did see, visiting their offices, or appearing at hearings) or imagine. Those they saw included people living because of dialysis or transplantation; those they were asked to imagine would be those who must die from their illness because they could not afford the treatment—the "needless deaths." The National Kidney Foundation, an alliance of laity and physicians that advocated for research and carried out service to patients (as it still does), lobbied in favor of a federal program, as did the recently formed National Association of Patients on Hemodialysis. Dialysis recipients spoke at hearings of the House Ways and Means Committee on November 4, 1971, and one, Shep Glazer, even had dialysis initiated before the committee, but it was terminated after a few minutes when he developed a cardiac arrhythmia (he recovered quickly). Nephrologists Belding Scribner and George Schreiner (the latter well positioned in Washington) provided clinical information and voiced the appeal from the kidney's growing body of medical specialists.

Acting together, these factors within and outside of Congress effected passage of the Medicare amendment that authorized what came to be called the End-Stage Renal Disease (ESRD) Program. It is of some interest to add that chronic kidney failure was made eligible for Medicare coverage by designating it a cause of *disability;* once again Bright's Disease was contemplated in relation to the capacity for work.[24] Since I've chosen to devote considerable attention in this book to the names, or diagnostic labels, given to kidney disease, "end-stage renal disease" warrants some comments. As with so many medical phrases, an abbreviation—ESRD—saves breath and time and in this case avoids speaking the painful word "end-stage." Nonetheless, the term recalls the ominous import of "Bright's Disease," but made explicit—"end-stage." ESRD arose as a bureaucratic category, a sort of disease defined by entitlement. It also can be understood as the kidney disease of having no kidneys, or no *working* kidneys, or maybe the disease of being treated for the absence of kidneys. As will be described later, it can claim its own, novel set of symptoms. ESRD is something of a reversion to the broadness of the old labels "dropsy" or "Bright's Disease," for once the kidneys have failed, ESRD is pretty much the same regardless of what caused the failure. That is, at that point, the precise diagnosis, perhaps selected painstakingly by biopsy from the arcane and ever-changing classification system, matters little.

Estimates of the costs for Medicare's ESRD program proved almost laughably conservative from the first, and the expenses have always far exceeded estimates. Although there have been efforts to reduce expenditures, there has been no retreat from the commitment to pay for dialysis and transplantation for virtually all Americans with terminal renal failure. In 2003 Medicare spent over $18 billion for care of persons with ESRD, about 14 billion of which paid for dialysis treatment, the remainder for kidney transplants. Private health insurance and patients themselves paid several billion more.[25]

PROVIDING MAINTENANCE DIALYSIS

Once the passage of P.L. 92-603 virtually eliminated ability to pay as a criterion for eligibility to receive chronic hemodialysis, facilities quickly expanded to accommodate more and more patients. Formation of proprietary dialysis treatment centers preceded passage of the funding measure, but it no doubt fueled the astounding growth of the for-profit dialysis industry in the United States.[26] Constantine Hampers, formerly a physician with the pioneering renal division of Peter Bent Brigham Hospital, and others in 1970 established their outpatient center in Boston and the corporation known as National Medical Care. By 1972 the company ran fifteen centers, and forty-eight by 1975. It became the dominant source of chronic dialytic care in Boston, Washington, D.C., Dallas, Philadelphia, and other cities. Although the affiliated or salaried physicians often held teaching positions at medical schools, the NMC units were usually freestanding and for-profit. Here was another invention, mercantile more than technologic: a nationwide commercial system for the efficient mass-provision of chronic hemodialysis, analogous to the national chains of retail stores, fast-food stops, and oil-change purveyors that came to dominate the American consumer market. NMC (later acquired by other companies with consequent changes of name) led the field, but local and regional commercial units also flourished, so that by 2000, for-profit enterprises carried out over 75 percent of hemodialysis for chronic outpatients in the United States. In 1980 Arnold Relman, nephrologist-turned-editor of the influential *New England Journal of Medicine,* trenchantly included this phenomenon in his essay called "The New Medical-Industrial Complex."[27]

The for-profit dialysis companies, which for the most part preceded the rise of commercial general hospitals, needless to say raised controversy. Should life-sustaining health care serve as a source of profit? To what extent did the profit contribute to the unexpectedly high cost to Medicare? Would the profit motive lead to treatment shortcuts? And, more specifically to ESRD care, did the proliferation of freestanding commercial dialysis centers inhibit the option of self-dialysis at home, which some authorities argued led to better rehabilitation and survival? Did the easy availability of dialysis centers reduce physicians' enthusiasm for the alternative and in many ways superior treatment for ESRD, transplantation? (Transplantation is the subject of chapter 8.) The physician leaders of NMC in turn argued that the efficiencies and economies of scale and the focus on doing one sort of job well kept costs down while sustaining the quality of care provided.[28] The intensity of the debate fluctuated over the years, while commercial dialysis operations grew in the United States and spread around the world.

In 1989 American nephrologists heard an unexpected and shocking revelation: data reported at a symposium in Dallas purported to show that American dialysis recipients lived less long and felt less well than those in Europe and Japan. That is, in the country where chronic dialysis began and grew rapidly into a huge American-style entrepreneurial system, its practitioners stood accused of not doing it very well.[29] At first, nephrologists in the United States posited—or assumed—that the inferior longevity merely reflected the inclusiveness of the national program, which welcomed old and medically complicated patients of the sort who might not have received treatment in England or Japan. Several critics within nephrology suggested that its training programs, so many of which emphasized physiological research, gave too little curricular attention to ESRD care, thus producing half-trained practitioners.[30] But neither of these explanations seemed adequate. An enormous effort arose to study and define "adequacy of dialysis," and particularly the mix of medical, economic, and behavioral determinants of dialysis *time,* meaning the duration of each of the thrice-weekly treatments—effectively, the dose of dialysis. In the nascent years of chronic dialysis, no one knew how many hours per week were needed to achieve something like well-being for the typical recipient, though Scribner attributed his initial success in the early 1960s to insisting on more rather than less. But in some centers the length of delivered treatment had declined during the 1980s, and the overall national average by then compared poorly with figures from other countries.

No party stood either wholly responsible for this deficiency, or entirely guiltless. As the cost of the ESRD program and profits to the proprietary companies both soared, in the early 1980s Medicare reduced reimbursements to all dialysis centers. Reduction in expenditures followed: staffing levels declined, and the suggestion certainly arose, never to be proved, that operators of the freestanding units also reduced duration of dialysis to allow for more treatments from each machine and thereby maintain profits. But even if true, it was not so simple. Some patients adhered poorly to their dialysis schedules, omitting visits or negotiating to conclude treatment before reaching the prescribed number of minutes.

This phenomenon occurred less frequently in other countries. The 1970s and 1980s had witnessed in the United States a growing assertion of patients' self-determination and autonomy within a movement that sought to adjust the power relationship between patient and doctor. It was linked to the rise of bioethics as an academic subdiscipline and a sort of paramedical specialty. The fifth, or even fourth, hour of hemodialysis becomes for many of those needing this treatment tedious almost beyond endurance, and for some brings muscle cramps or other symptoms: patients claimed and exercised the right to "sign off" the machine whenever in the treatment they wished. While relatively few did so often or irresponsibly, over a month or a year someone might end up deficient in total dialysis dose, especially if the amount prescribed was barely enough. To the dialysis nurse fell the difficult job of convincing the patient to stay put until completion of the full treatment, though she or he was the one who most had to watch the misery and hear the complaints. In short, from the budget offices in Washington to the person in the chair at a neighborhood dialysis center, an array of social and medical circumstances favored a subtle but important shrinkage of treatment time, with potential for deterioration in the quality of dialytic care. As more information accumulated in the 1990s, nephrologists restored the length of dialysis treatments and adopted technological improvements to increase the dose.[31]

From a broader perspective, one might say that patients, clinicians, managers, and anyone else involved with maintenance dialysis were working out the limits and tolerances in this particular new relationship between human being and machine. Establishing such limits, particularly determining optimally how long a human being and a machine should interact, has been a recurring need of the industrial age, beginning perhaps most obviously with the railroad locomotive and train in the mid-nineteenth century. Physicians and others weighed the undoubted benefit of the novel and swift form of travel against the assault of vibration and noise endured by drivers and passengers for hours at a time.[32] For television, a machine whose career progressed concurrently with that of the artificial kidney, debate continues over how long persons, particularly children, should sit attached to it. For the man or woman with ESRD, of course, to live demands the coupling of human and machine, unlike the optional relationship with television—which some in fact consider life-draining. Still, for the person on dialysis, time on the machine, measured to the minute, became a ruling medical and moral determination.

The troubling (to some) issue of corporate profit motive sharpened another debate—should this life-extending care be offered to persons with dementia, disabling systemic diseases, or advanced age? Would persons who might not "benefit" (the word was often used and rarely defined) from dialysis, and possibly only endure lengthier end-of-life suffering, occupy chairs in order to keep the shifts filled? Or, might in time those not truly "end-stage" find themselves being dialyzed? Whereas some mistakes and abuses must have occurred, no one seriously accused dialysis units or nephrologists of dragging unwilling, or full-kidneyed patients, to the machine. Such means of filling the chairs would have been superfluous in any case, for ESRD in the 1970s and beyond appeared to be more widespread than anyone had imagined, rightly looked upon as an "epidemic."[33] Whereas the earliest select patients of Seattle tended to be young and white, with disease limited to the kidneys, the epidemic of the 1970s and 1980s sent (as will be described in more detail in the following chapters) increasing numbers of older, especially black, Americans to dialysis units, their kidneys destroyed most often by a pernicious combination of diabetes and hypertension. Since many such men and women were among the urban and uninsured poor, the combination of a unique governmental benefit program and the rapid growth of the commercial units fortuitously avoided what otherwise would have been a provocative test of social equity and an intolerable burden on inner-city hospitals. Whatever might be the objections to for-profit dialysis, or for-profit health care in general, National Medical Care and the other large companies had the capital to build and the wherewithal to deliver artificial kidney treatments in the hundreds of thousands.

CHRONIC DIALYSIS IN THE UNITED KINGDOM

The eminent British nephrologist and historian of medicine J. Stewart Cameron provides a thoughtful analysis of the slow acceptance of chronic dialysis in the United Kingdom in his book on the history of hemodialysis.[34] Since 1948, the National Health Service (NHS) has provided medical care to virtually all Britons, and—though there are failings in such a system—has done so effectively and efficiently. The portion of the British gross national product devoted to health care has been, for better or worse, lower than that in most Western European nations and much less than that in the United States. Maintenance dialysis, with its requirement for indefinite provision of labor-intensive technological care, not surprisingly, challenged the philosophy and fairness of the British system.

Nephrologists initiated dialysis for chronic cases in the early

1960s in London, Newcastle, Edinburgh, and Birmingham, though considerable objection appeared in the British medical press. The opposition centered on concerns about utilization of resources and also on the problem of transmission of hepatitis within dialysis units, which for unknown reasons occurred more often in the United Kingdom than elsewhere. Some American renal specialists had also voiced skepticism about expansion of maintenance dialysis in the United States, questioning whether the process had been adequately tested and proved.[35] In 1965, the British Department of Health convened a committee to look into the question of maintenance dialysis, and the outcome was a recommendation to establish a limited network of regional renal units to provide dialysis and transplantation. The NHS had thirty-two operating by 1970. In determining which sort of persons with irreversible kidney failure might qualify for such care, the British chose the word "suitability," but with the same intent as the American concept of "who might benefit." Indeed, initial criteria included younger age, absence of systemic (i.e., nonkidney) disease, and stable home environment, similar to those adopted by the early American programs. Although the parallels are far from perfect, so far, little differed from the story in the United States—a few people started on treatment by interested nephrologists in several locations, a commissioned report, and support by the national government of something like a pilot program comprising a set number of centers.

But then, the stories do diverge, for a complexity of reasons. Hepatitis outbreaks within dialysis units continued to dampen enthusiasm in Great Britain. But more important, as suggested by Cameron and others, were economic and what one might call cultural factors. The care of ESRD never became a discreet, funded program within the NHS, with assurance of coverage to all deemed medically eligible; rather, centrally or regionally, administrators each year had to consider all medical needs of the population and make difficult choices about where expenditures would go. Care of renal disease competed with other requirements. In this circumstance, chronic dialysis stagnated from 1970 until the 1980s, when availability improved. Although patients in the United Kingdom much more than in the United States employed the less expensive modes of dialysis at home, and kidney transplantation, statistics revealed that Britain showed sharply lower rates of providing care for terminal renal failure than most other nations of Western Europe.

And yet, surprisingly, renal units in the United Kingdom during the 1970s and 1980s often saw some of their capacity going unused. In the British system, referral for specialty care within the NHS almost always channels through the general practitioner, and some failed to send people who might have been eligible. Dialysis apparently was perceived for a long time as even less available than it was, and also as something exotic within the national culture of medicine. Low expectations, presumably of both general practitioners and patients, limited the intensity of political pressure placed on the NHS to expand renal care; the failure to build more units in turn maintained the sense of scarce access. Critics have applied the term "covert rationing" to the outcome of this dynamic, covert because the NHS never actually prescribed the number of chronic dialysis recipients that would be accommodated nationally, or within any one region.

In this regard, neither the United States nor the United Kingdom has engaged in much central, rational planning for the care of end-stage kidney disease. The NHS for the most part allowed things to sort themselves as best they might at the local level, looking the other way as older (but not necessarily decrepit) patients failed to find their way to treatment. Medicare in the United States, on the other hand (through congressional action) committed to paying for the treatment of effectively all patients with kidney failure, including the frail and demented, and dealt with the exploding costs by simply lowering, then fixing, the fee paid per treatment. In thinking historically about the two systems, two questions occur, at least to this writer. First, how decisive was the role of for-profit dialytic care in the United States in ensuring widespread, or even excessive, availability? Of course, such an enterprise could not have arisen in Great Britain. And second, why did the idea of the "identifiable" life and the "needless death," so persuasive to sensibilities in the United States, not enter into debates about the support of dialysis in the United Kingdom?

—⟨∞⟩—

A Later Perspective

The typical chronic dialysis recipient of 2006 reports for three treatments weekly, each lasting three to four hours. This plan generally allows for adequate removal of retained toxins and fluid, so long as everything is functioning properly. A key determinant of success is the status of the person's "access to the circulation." Optimally, this will be a fistula, a surgical connection of an artery and vein created usually in the arm as one approaches the need for dialysis. When an artery is joined to a vein, the higher arterial pressure causes the vein to enlarge and thicken: this allows for repeated puncture and insertion of the needles that will deliver blood flow to the artificial kidney. An unaltered vein will not yield enough flow. The external shunt is now rarely used. It served well in its day but, being partly in and partly out of the bloodstream, was subject to clotting and infection. When a person's veins are small, a synthetic vessel (graft) can be surgically sewn between an artery and vein and serve as the access, though it usually proves more subject to clotting than a fistula. For immediate or short-term use, or when no other access can be achieved, a plastic indwelling catheter into a large vein will work but again proves vulnerable to infection and clotting. Perhaps nothing is more essential to the well-being of someone on dialysis than a well-functioning fistula.

With the recognition in the 1980s that survival statistics for U.S. dialysis recipients seemed inferior to those elsewhere, a large effort was begun to determine more precisely how "adequacy" of dialysis could be measured and optimized, really a question of dosing. The amount of effective dialysis one receives depends upon the amount of time on the machine, the quantity of blood flow, the size and attributes of the dialysis filter, and the flow of the dialysate. The dialysate (not the best term, but long in use) is the physiological fluid caused to flow on the side of the membrane opposite the patient's blood flow. Urea, creatinine, potassium, phosphate, and other substances will move by "gradient diffusion" from the blood into the dialysate, which is discarded. The overall effectiveness of the system is now measured using certain calculations, either the "urea reduction ratio" or "KT/V urea." As with much else in twenty-first century medicine, "practice guidelines" have been established (though still much debated) against which a patient's measurements can be compared. Recently, considerable enthusiasm has arisen, more in Europe but now also in North America, for daily dialysis carried out overnight. There may be important gains in well-being and survival with this plan, though of course it can add expense and inconvenience.

All dialysis recipients require a variety of medications, either consumed as pills or administered during the dialytic treatments. These include: drugs for high blood pressure; "phosphate binders" to reduce absorption in the intestine of phosphate from food (dialysis is not very good at removing phosphate); vitamin D and other vitamins; and the blood-forming substance epoetin (which is discussed in chapter 7). Why so many drugs? The kidneys participate in the regulation of the body's blood pressure, and most chronic renal disease leads to hypertension. The organs as well carry out several activities related to the adjustment of calcium and phosphorus in the body, including the final step in the manufacture of vitamin D. Dialysis does not replace these functions. Left untreated, the changes in calcium and phosphorus (and their regulatory substance, parathyroid hormone) can lead to thinning of bones, bone pain, and even fractures. Even adverse effects of calcium on the heart and blood vessels may occur.

Medicare's ESRD program in the United States continues its struggle to limit expenditures. Its main strategy has been to simply avoid any increase in the fee paid for the dialytic treatments themselves, but it cannot restrict the number of persons entering maintenance care. It has, however, agreed to pay for the injections of epoetin, which are given during dialysis, one or more times per week for most people. These payments have accounted for some of the sharpest increases in Medicare's outlay for renal care.[36]

Because of the limits on how much a given dialysis treatment can do, patients must limit ingestions of fluid and usually should follow some dietary restrictions. In order to maintain good nutritional status and muscle mass, chronic dialysis recipients are encouraged to eat protein—quite the opposite of advice they may have received before beginning dialysis—but some limitation of foods high in salt, potassium, and phosphate is still requested.

CHAPTER SEVEN

Coupled to the Artificial Kidney

—~~~—

The conventional history of medicine from time to time offers troubling stories of new therapies tried out on powerless or even oppressed members of society. One thinks of surgeon J. Marion Sims's perfection of the operation for vesicovaginal fistula on slave women in nineteenth-century Alabama, or in the twentieth century, of "psychosurgery" (frontal lobotomy) for the treatment of institutionalized patients with mental disease. In neither of these customary examples do the practitioners stand accused of malice, and, as it happens, at least some of those first subjected to the treatments, and their successors, gained benefit. The earliest application of the artificial kidney for treating terminal chronic renal disease attracted much controversy, as we have seen, precisely because it was applied mostly to middle-class, white men—those in Western society considered empowered and entitled. This innovation occurred, however, in the twentieth-century environment of "modern medicine" and the unprecedented confidence in scientific and technological advance as the means to securing health. Though termed experimental by some skeptics within the nephrology community, chronic dialysis managed to skip some steps and garner the epithet "life-saving" at its first appearance.

FROM THE FEW TO MANY

Few in number, the early chronic hemodialysis recipients achieved a degree of status as celebrities, or at least as public figures. Belding Scribner's first patient, Clyde Shields, became the subject of a short film, and his photograph has appeared in many historical accounts of dialysis. As noted in chapter 6, Shep Glazer, who did his dialysis at home in Brooklyn, undertook to demonstrate the process on himself in front of a congressional committee. Several other male dialysis patients at one unit in Brooklyn, including a lawyer and a recent graduate of Columbia University, formed the National Association of Patients on Hemodialysis (now the National Association of Kidney Patients). They campaigned to win governmental support for dialysis in the United States. *A Chance to Live,* a "photo-essay" about chronic dialysis published by the Kidney Disease Control Program of the U.S. Department of Health, Education, and Welfare in 1968 leaves its subjects (most, but not all, white men) anonymous but depicts them as quiet heroes, some managing their own treatments, some sustaining a full family and work life despite their ESRD.[1]

In fact, their lives did display quiet valor (and for many people on dialysis, still do), even if they did no more than just carry on. The early patients were described as showing considerable "*esprit de corps.*"[2] They were, and some of them knew they were, as much pioneers in a strange new endeavor as their physicians and nurses, some very actively so. Those who chose to dialyze at home had to learn a great deal and master a complex set of skills, and in exchange enjoyed much more control of their time and schedules than those who reported on shift to centers.[3] Occasionally someone would relocate to a new community in order to get treated at a particular dialysis unit.[4] Many patients outside urban centers travel considerable distances by car or van three times each week to obtain their treatments. Taking the machine home, or (rarely) changing homes, or sometimes driving forty miles for each visit to a center, these individuals with renal disease joined many other historical and contemporaneous persons with chronic illness in search of a cure—pilgrims to the healing shrines of saints, consumptives to the sanitaria, the hay feverish to mountain resorts, the dropsical to warmer climates. Even those not doing dialysis at home came to experience chronic dialysis as something like a job (as we will explore later in the chapter). Thus, as their doctors helped establish the new medical subspecialty of nephrology, those indefinitely coupled to the artificial kidney in effect constituted a new specialty of *patient*. Some, who served as leaders in organizations or columnists for the groups' publications, or spokespersons in their units, indeed became something like professional patients. Such activities, combining service to others with enhanced self-esteem, of course continue to the present day.[5]

There are many to be served: as already noted in chapter 6, the few dialysis recipients of the 1960s have grown to well over 325,000 in the United States and probably nearly one million in the world as this is written. In the United States, over 90 percent of these people receive hemodialysis, while 8 percent carry out the alternative treatment of peritoneal dialysis at home, sometimes overnight using an automated device.[6] They have changed qualitatively as well. The earliest patients were mostly under age fifty and relatively free of disease other than the loss of their renal function from a malady purely located in the kidneys—usually glomerular nephritis (née Bright's Disease).[7] The very first participants in Scribner's program were white, which is itself not surprising since in 1960 not many African Americans lived in Seattle. Today (2005–2006), about 20 percent of Americans on dialysis have passed their seventy-fifth birthday, and eighty-year-olds represent the fastest-growing segment of the hemodialysis population. Whereas the presence of diabetes excluded patients in the tentative early period of chronic hemodialysis, now over 40 percent of those in the U.S. ESRD program (and many elsewhere in the world) have lost their kidney function at least in part from this destructive disorder of sugar metabolism.

Described as epidemic in the industrial world, diabetes and "diabetic nephropathy" warrant some further discussion here. The advent of insulin treatment in the 1920s changed juvenile diabetes (now called "insulin-dependent" or type 1) from a disease that usually led to death by the teenage or early adult years into a chronic ailment. The welcome gain in life span with insulin, however, provides enough time for several of the now-familiar complications of diabetes to develop, particularly visual loss from retinopathy and kidney failure with proteinuria from "diabetic glomerulopathy."[8] Nonetheless, diabetic renal disease seemed comparatively rare in the 1960s and early 1970s, winning only a few pages in the early nephrology textbooks of this period. Somehow, by the 1980s it seemed to be everywhere. No one factor adequately explains this unexpected burden. Many of those with diabetic renal disease have "maturity onset," or type 2, diabetes, and the fierce proliferation of this disease in the late twentieth century can be assigned, if only in part, to rising rates of overeating, inactivity, and obesity.[9] Diabetic nephropathy became the Bright's Disease of the later twentieth-century industrial world. Bright and the nineteenth century saw the renal malady of their day as rooted in social circumstance (poor workers soaked and chilled on the job) and depraved self-indulgence—drunkenness. Though a genetic component plays a role, the dominant cause of renal failure of the twentieth century seems an artifact of *its* society's ill-chosen ways of living. And the wages of such sinning pile up: because of the deterioration of blood vessels and circulation that diabetes causes, diabetics who are on dialysis tend to have problems with their access (the modified or synthetic blood vessel used for connection to the dialysis device), frequent hospitalizations, and shorter lives than ESRD patients without diabetes.

"Dr. Owen, ain't it nothing but black folks on dialysis?" a Boston patient asked nephrologist William F. Owen in 1992, presumably after looking around the dialysis unit, and Dr. Owen used the question to begin an article reviewing the differences in the frequency of renal disease between persons of color and whites, and the onerous consequences within African-American communities.[10] There are overall more white Americans on dialysis, but the *rate* of ESRD is (as previously noted) three to four times higher for blacks. Since American medical care mirrors American society, the segregation of cities along with the disproportionate representation of kidney failure among African Americans can certainly make the Bostonian's question understandable.

Indeed, patterns of segregation may have even made it difficult for the professional nephrology community to recognize this "racial disparity," to use a phrase that is very current as I write this. But the disparity was apparent to all by the 1980s and led the National Institutes of Health in the United States to undertake a large investigation called the African American Study of Kidney Disease and Hypertension (AASK) in 1990. It sought to determine whether any class of drug for treating hypertension would, in blacks, prove more effective than others in preventing the kidney disorder referred to as "hypertensive nephrosclerosis."[11] This is the dominant cause of ESRD among blacks, though rates of diabetes are also high, so that high blood pressure and diabetes provide a doubly destructive influence on the kidneys. In addition, in the United States the glomerular disease called focal segmental glomerulosclerosis (FSGS) occurs mainly among African Americans and often leads to ESRD. Why persons of color (and other minority groups as well) seem unusually vulnerable to failure of the kidneys remains unknown but constitutes an area of much research as this is written. Medical scientists naturally look for genetic or other biological explanations, but access to care and other socioeconomic variables also have been considered.[12]

Whatever the reasons for so much ESRD among blacks in the United States and elsewhere, "going to dialysis" is nearly as familiar a part of African-American life in the cities as is going to church.[13] Both the American Kidney Fund and the National Kidney Foundation, the large national service and education organizations concerned with kidney disease, initiated special programs aimed at black Americans. Yet, at least as reflected in the popular African-American periodicals through 2005, little awareness of renal failure as a particular affliction of blacks seemed to exist within African-American communities, though a considerable number of pages are given to its main causes, high blood pressure and diabetes.[14] (As will be seen in chapter 8, the prevalence of kidney disease among blacks occasionally becomes visible in the popular press through stories of celebrity transplantations.) Already linked to the painful genetic disorder sickle-cell anemia, and discovered to be at high risk for prostate cancer and glaucoma, perhaps African-Americans neither want nor need further self-identification with diseases.[15] As suggested at the beginning of this chapter, the federal ESRD program and the growth of freestanding dialysis centers at least have provided access to dialysis treatment or kidney transplantation for the numerous poor and unemployed inner-city blacks in the United States. But it is a painful irony of American health care that some working but uninsured Americans cannot afford the blood pressure medications and medical visits that might enable them to avoid eventually joining the ranks of those who "go to dialysis," the costs of which *will* be "covered."

We can summarize this way: after fifty years of chronic dialysis (in the United States), the numbers are huge and comprise persons of every age, tint, and ethnic background. But the face of the dialysis recipient has changed. It is no longer that of forty-year-old white men—those dialyzed with the first Seattle shunts, those coming from New York to lobby Congressmen, or those pictured in the cheerful pages of the 1968 U.S. Public Health Service publication *A Chance to Live.* Rather, it is the graying African-American woman who looks forthrightly at the reader from the cover of *Diabetes and Chronic Kidney Disease,* a 2004 educational pamphlet of the National Kidney Foundation.

THE EXPERIENCE OF DIALYSIS

A diagnosis of Bright's Disease, as recounted in earlier chapters, acquired a fearful reputation and came to an ill person and family almost as a sentence of death. Needless to say, the phrase "end-stage renal disease" conveys a similar meaning. "Possibly the name is most frightening, end stage renal disease," wrote a woman in Georgia in the 1980s. "It sounds like the end of the world. That's the way I felt [upon first learning of it]. I cried and cried."[16] "When I was diagnosed I cried like a baby," said an African American in Rochester, New York, in 1995. "I was devastated. I thought this meant I would never see my grandchildren grow up."[17] For many of those facing chronic dialysis, fear of the disease transforms to fear of the treatment, which itself is imagined as the pathway to death. During discussions of the approaching need for dialysis, my patients seemed to always report knowing someone who started on dialysis, "but he didn't last long." Nonetheless, with the amazing resilience so often seen in persons dealing with chronic illness, the weeping ends, and life—now with the machine—goes on.

Then, to be sure, the vast majority of dialysis recipients show up for their treatments regularly (a few do them at home), feel tolerably well at least some of the time, and are glad to be alive. A tiny minority are not and after some interval voluntarily withdraw from chronic dialysis, choosing death. This comes, of course, as a sad and difficult event for all involved. Family members and professional caregivers struggle to judge how forcefully they can and should oppose the patient's decision.[18] Some persons who are on dialysis, sometimes after a long wait, receive a kidney transplantation, and—if all goes well—elevate toward that status called "cure," a phrase that for many years has known far more use by fund-raisers than by physicians.

Chronic dialysis is not a *cure*. The artificial kidney, even after decades of refinement, remains in the early twenty-first century still a paltry imitation of the real thing, especially when employed for only twelve or so hours weekly (the real ones do not take time off). Thus, it achieves only an incomplete restoration of health. In fact, the dialysis patient has been referred to as a "marginal man," suspended between the world of the well and the world of the sick.[19] Nephrologist and longtime dialysis recipient Peter Lundin expressed it this way in 1990: "There is still a sense of weakness, a sense of being ill. And then there is the overall sense of well-being. Now I certainly can say that during most of those 24 years I have felt well, but most of the time you really do not have the sense of feeling normal, of feeling healthy."[20]

Others on dialysis have written about the symptoms they feel despite optimal treatment. "Before my system adjusted to dialysis," wrote newspaperman Lee Foster in 1976, "I developed common unpleasant symptoms—cramps, dizzy spells, intense itching, a feeling sometimes of being unable to catch my breath, even terrible searing heartburn and hiccups from my medications."[21] Most of these symptoms relented, but for some people mysterious phenomena like itching persist. "I had a lot of side effects, a lot of difficulty with the machine, discomfort—itching particularly—constant itching that was the worst discomfort," one interviewee reported for an article published in 1980.[22] Others are never troubled by itching but suffer painful muscle cramps during or shortly after some of their treatments. Still others experience pain in the bones or joints. A general lack of energy limits some individuals,

while others feel literally "washed out" and wiped out mostly during the several hours immediately following each treatment.

For many men and women receiving long-term dialysis, thirst
remains a nagging symptom and source of frustration. Persons
with ESRD eventually cease excreting any urine, so most of the
fluid ingested, be it water, coffee, beer, cola, or juice, must be removed at the thrice-weekly dialytic treatments. The machine has
a large capacity to remove excess water from the body at any one
treatment, but "taking off" too much at one session can induce
symptomatic or even dangerous drops in a patient's blood pressure, as well as nausea or cramps. Thus, it's necessary to avoid
taking in large quantities of fluid during the intervals between
treatments. "Resisting fluid is not so easy," said Lee Foster, the
New York Times writer. "The Sunday of the last Super Bowl game,
for example, was disastrous. We were invited to a house party
in the country. There was a heaping buffet and a well-stocked
bar. I lost all control, stuffed myself with forbidden salty foods
. . . drank glasses of water, cider, and ginger ale. I gained eleven
pounds."[23] Many memoirists of life with the machine comment
on the struggle to *not drink*. Regrettably, to make matters worse,
many on dialysis in fact suffer from exaggerated thirst. An article
titled "Patient Perceptions of the Hemodialysis Regimen," in the
bleakly named journal *Loss, Grief and Care,* turns out to center entirely on thirst.[24] It may be recalled that medical writers had once
deemed excessive thirst a characteristic symptom of the disease
"dropsy."

Even in 2005, forty-five years since the advent of chronic dialysis, an article in the *Journal of the American Society of Nephrology*
revealed a continuing high rate of bothersome symptoms among
dialysis recipients. Notably frequent were tiredness, dry skin, itching, and pain felt in bones or joints.[25] On the other hand, those
manifestations of seriously diseased kidneys first pointed out by
Richard Bright and later called uremia, such as vomiting, seizures,
inflammatory pain around the heart (pericarditis), for the most
part do not occur in patients receiving reasonably adequate dialysis treatments. Why, then, do so many not feel more well, more
of the time? The muscle cramps and transient feelings of nausea
during the treatments are something like immediate side effects

of the therapy itself. Other symptoms, like pains originating in bones or joints, represent very slowly developing consequences of renal failure that patients did not live long enough to feel until dialysis became available. That is, the bone pains can result from one of several complex disorders of the skeleton related to loss of the kidney's ability to properly adjust the content of calcium and phosphorus in the body. But before dialysis, persons with kidneys so impaired as to lose this ability did not live long enough for the bone problem to reach a symptomatic phase. In a sense, then, ESRD is a disease different from uremia; it is more the disease of dialysis than the disease of sick kidneys. Many of the symptoms people on dialysis endure are possible, paradoxically, only through staying alive by way of dialysis.

Another example is the anemia (lack of enough red cells in the blood) of renal failure. The kidneys, quite aside from their excretory functions, produce a blood-forming hormone called erythropoietin and thereby regulate the quantity of red cells, the oxygen-carrying elements of blood. No convincing theories have arisen to explain why the kidneys, in an evolutionary sense, acquired this odd job. In any case, as any form of chronic kidney disease worsens, the kidneys lose capacity to make erythropoietin, production of red cells in the bone marrow slows down, and anemia results. It is in good part the anemia that accounts for the fatigue and lack of energy sensed by many persons with ESRD. But, before dialysis or kidney transplantation, persons with failing kidneys usually died before the anemia itself became a major contributor to their lack of well-being. In the late 1980s, a synthetic form of erythropoietin became available for injection, offering what nephrologists hoped would amount to a revolution in the care and well-being of their dialysis patients. Indeed, various clinical trials and the experiences of most dialysis units did show that on the whole, people gained a brisker sense of well-being and higher exercise tolerance once their anemia had been improved by epoetin-alpha, as the new agent was called. Epoetin-alpha, often shortened to EPO, stands among the first major successes of "recombinant," or genetically produced, drugs and also represents one of the first instances of patenting a sequence of DNA. Yet, as noted above, studies published in 2005 still found that many individuals on dialysis suffered from a sense of fatigue and lack of energy, even after improvement of their anemia.[26]

The developer and manufacturer of epoetin-alpha, Amgen Corporation of Thousand Oaks, California, released the drug in conjunction with a massive undertaking of promotion and education, and, as with many drugs, it came to be referred to and prescribed by its trade name, Epogen. Amgen representatives helped facilitate payment by insurers or Medicare for the costly injections and helped some patients with no coverage obtain the agent. The company achieved extraordinary financial success: in 1990 *Fortune* magazine named Epogen its "product of the year," and by 1992 Amgen total sales exceeded $1 billion.[27] Amgen has become (at least in the United States) a major patron of nephrology. Its support of local and national conferences, and its gaudy presence at annual association meetings (including painting shuttle buses Amgen yellow), display another facet of the vast economic interlinkage of medicine, government, and industry in the large-scale care of people with irreversible failure of the kidneys.

GETTING BACK TO WORK, OR IS DIALYSIS THE JOB?

In earlier chapters, I pointed out that several of the "renal physicians" encountered in this book tended to think about the treatment of persons with chronic Bright's Disease in terms of keeping the patient working, or getting him back to work, at least when treating men. It was perhaps not until the twentieth century, with the sharp reduction in death rates from acute infectious diseases, that medicine had formulated the concept of chronic disease and recognized its importance. The very idea of chronic disease as a category arose in relation to disability—meaning the inability to go to work. One of the early and prominent writers on the subject, Ernst Boas of New York City, in his 1940 book *The Unseen Plague: Chronic Disease,* wrote: "The chief aim of treatment of the chronic disabilities, in which complete restitution to normal can no longer be expected, is to arrest the progress of the disease, and to enable the patient to maintain or resume his accustomed place in society and in his family. The patient must be taught to regard his illness not as the focus of his life, but as a handicap to be overcome. All too often a patient is advised to quit work and to devote his whole time to his cure, when it would be far better to keep him at his occupation."[28]

We can recall from chapter 4 Thomas Addis's belief in the primacy of work, and that the physician caring for patients with chronic Bright's Disease must try to "keep them on the firing line to the very last gasp."[29] As also suggested earlier, the *worth* of a man has long been equated with the *work* of a man, especially within modern industrial society. It may also be remembered that the federal ESRD payment program in the United States was created by declaring those with kidney failure to be disabled and thus eligible for Medicare. Paradoxically, the early favorable publicity given to dialytic care portrayed it as a treatment that would enable a person with uremia to resume employment. That this would occur as a matter of course entered forcefully into the rhetoric of legislators and others pressing for a federal program—dialysis would allow people with renal disease to work and earn rather than require support.[30] And ever since, "rehabilitation," understood as going back to work, has been to a greater or lesser extent—now lesser more than greater—an objective in the care of renal patients, as well as a measurement of the "success" of chronic dialysis.[31]

Writing about their lives with dialysis, patients often expressed their desire to work, the frustration felt when confronting the inability to return to a job, or the satisfaction of returning to productive activity in either the outside workplace or the home:[32]

> So, I liked my job, I enjoyed working. I wish I was healthy, I could still work, because I met a lot of nice people and it was nice. And, you have to quit your job because of this!

> The main reason I chose HHD [hemodialysis at home] was that it would allow me to continue to work, since my dialysis facility did not have an evening shift. I worked for the first 15 years on dialysis. This allowed me to remain a contributing member of society and gave meaning to my life.

> Patient rehabilitation and work frequently conflict with the dialysis center's schedule, which is designed to meet the needs of the professional staff. Many patients accept their shift assign-

ment and do not insist on scheduling that would allow them to
work.

Since returning to full-time work I have felt much better physi-
cally and mentally although the more disciplined existence can
be overtaxing when difficulties with dialysis occur. Many dialysis
patients do not work at all and often become depressed and in-
trospective.

Today I manage my house (with some help I admit), stay very
active with my children and my husband, participate actively in
our church, work part-time selling Avon, and serve on several
committees related to ESRD.

In the United States, the requirements of the Social Security
system reduce or eliminate subsidy payments if a recipient exceeds
a certain level of earned income (coverage of ESRD care itself is
not affected). Since many on dialysis have come from the ranks of
low-wage earners, they would sometimes risk losing income, already small, by going back to work, even if they felt strong enough
to do so:[33]

> If you don't do anything, you can get help. But if you want to
> work and you want to pull your weight, you can't get any help.
> That is the problem.

> If only I could make at least two-thirds of what I'll be receiving
> from Social Security disability insurance, I would like to work.

Not surprisingly, hemodialysis patients have often described
being a hemodialysis patient as *itself* a job. This realization would
seem obvious for those individuals choosing to do their dialysis
(hemo- or peritoneal) at home, a complex and demanding set of
tasks. Yet for some of these, it becomes their *second* job, since they
might have elected home dialysis in order to schedule treatments
so as to allow work during the day. But even for dialysis recipients
who report three times weekly to a center—the vast majority of
persons with ESRD—the activity does own some attributes of a
job: one has to repeatedly show up on schedule, at a place outside
the home, to pass a series of hours in a manner not particularly
interesting or enjoyable:[34]

Sometimes I dread getting up at five-thirty a.m., making the forty-six mile trip [to the dialysis clinic], but it's like going to a job. People must work to live and I need my machine to live.

[*"Raymond" looks at dialysis like a job,"* states a reporter.] You get up, go to the dialysis center, and get it over with. I guess that I look at it as a necessary part of my life—nothing more and nothing less.

Thomas Addis had advised his patient Linus Pauling and other patients to "forget about" their Bright's Disease—follow the diet, ignore the dropsy of the legs if not too marked, and pursue life and work. Persons on dialysis attempt to do something like this as best they can but find it difficult when the treatment has become their occupation.[35]

—◦◦◦—

Maintenance hemodialysis for persons who have irretrievably lost kidney function thus proves time consuming, constraining, and—at least for some—incompletely restorative. The proportion of patients able to work at a paying job has disappointed everyone involved at least since the inception of the ESRD program in the United States. The hope that improved stamina gained through the use of epoetin to improve anemia has been partly fulfilled, but other medical and particularly socioeconomic factors still have limited the likelihood of chronic hemodialysis recipients returning to work.[36] Not mentioned so far in this chapter is the episodic need for stays in the hospital to deal with a failure of the dialysis access (fistula or catheter), or to care for some complication of the treatment, the underlying renal failure, or a concurrent disease such as diabetes

CHRONIC HEMODIALYSIS AS SUCCESS AND FAILURE

In the United States, if not other parts of the world, the success of chronic hemodialysis in one sense has ensured its failure in another. Technical improvements and cumulating clinical know-how have made possible the care of older and more medically complex persons with kidney failure. A woman with slowly progressive chronic renal disease whom I help look after medically is scheduled to begin dialysis soon at age ninety. The establishment of a federal payment program and the flourishing of both commercial and noncommercial dialysis networks eliminated scarcity of resources as a variable. While better dialytic membranes and the invention of epoetin allowed many to feel better, countless others entered the dialysis unit with their bodies already worn down by the effects of diabetes, narrowed atherosclerotic arteries, heart disease, or simply age. As of the early twenty-first century, almost half of Americans on dialysis are over sixty-five years of age, with the mean age inching toward and beyond the point of normal retirement. Many young, black persons from the inner city, victims of renal failure from extreme hypertension or FSGS, entered dialysis while experiencing unemployment and an already poor quality of life: the artificial kidney could hardly be expected to make matters better for them. In short, going to work became increasingly meaningless as an epidemiological measurement of dialysis effectiveness (though hardly so for many individuals).

By the early 1990s, a movement had arisen to achieve a "redefinition of renal rehabilitation and its goals" as something more flexible than "return to productive employment." One suggested definition was "restoring the individual with disease or disability to optimal functioning in his or her own normal societal environment," whatever that might mean.[37] A vast amount of research since the 1980s has attempted to define what constitutes optimal medical and technical care of persons with ESRD. Such research uses as the "outcome" measure simply years of survival on dialysis: renal physicians since the 1990s rarely even talk about their patients getting back to work (dialysis social workers still do). Yet, some younger patients *do,* despite all obstacles, manage to perform some of life's work—be it teaching mathematics at college (and grading papers during dialysis), filling odd shifts as a security guard, practicing medicine, huckstering Amway distributorships, doing home repairs, managing family and household, even starting small businesses.[38] They do so for economic reasons, and to draw their sense of self and identity away from the machine and back to themselves. For some, the effort must be seen as a gallant triumph within the moral expectations and choices of maintenance hemodialysis.

Moral expectations? I have suggested in earlier sections of this book that the experience of disease, especially serious disease, usually reveals moral meanings of some sort. For the chronic hemodialysis recipient, each day offers opportunities to display strength and resolve, or the opposite—imperfect fulfillment of the role of "good patient." Here are reflections of four dialysis patients:[39]

> Carrying around an extra four kilograms of fluid [from drinking too much between treatments] is a lot. I hate feeling like that. Now I push myself to do something. Mentally I don't want to get down. I don't want to go back to where I was. I don't know what you call it? Willpower? The nurses here sometimes think I don't care, but that's not true.

> Challenges in life scream out for self-discipline. This is a factor that causes us to win, overcome, or lose. . . . When I first went on the dialysis machine, I accepted it as a personal challenge and an opportunity to use the self-discipline I had built during the years. . . . I have found the limitation of liquids to be very trying.

> Do I cheat on my diet? Of course I do, being only human. But I know how to cheat cautiously and creatively. Hardest of all to resist is taking a good long drink whenever I want to.

> You have to be patient, you have to be disciplined. I take it seriously. I've never missed a session . . . the life is hard, but what are you going to do about it? [This statement is from Patricia LeBlack, a Guyana-born British woman who in 2006 was in her thirty-ninth year of chronic dialysis, making her quite likely at the time the longest-surviving dialysis patient in the world.]

So the person receiving maintenance hemodialysis must continuously decide how well to do the job—to appear for all treatments, comply with the restrictions, contain desire, monitor limits, keep going to stay alive. That is, she or he contends daily with what the Greeks called *akrasia,* acting against one's best interest, or a lack of self-control. The rejection of appetite in favor of a higher good has been, of course, a teaching of major religions, not just dialysis doctors, nurses, and nutritionists.[40] As seen in three of the comments quoted above (and many similar statements could be added), the need for ascetic self-restraint centers particularly on one of the most profound biological drives known to human beings, the desire to drink water.

Patients know that in the moral setting of the dialysis unit, punishment will follow cheating: breath-robbing dropsy, then the tormenting cramps and faintness when the overburden of fluid has to be drained from the body during one treatment lasting three or four hours. Some suffer as well the added burden of guilt and self-reproach; and they risk loss of an approving and supportive attitude from nurses, physicians, and other staff. Of course, some small number of dialysis recipients simply behave in foolish and self-destructive ways, raising havoc for themselves, their families, and their treatment centers. It is worth repeating that most transcend their circumstances to resume at least some aspects of normal lives, and many even serve others, particularly in patients' organizations.

As I reread what I have written so far for this chapter, I find I have dealt with chronic hemodialysis more critically than I had intended, almost deriding or scolding it for its imperfections (as did anthropologist Alonzo Plough in his book from 1986 titled *Borrowed Time*).[41] The artificial kidney does, after all, keep alive something like one million persons throughout the world who have permanently lost the function of a major, indispensable organ, usually through no fault of their own. But it does not cure, and it misses qualifying fully as medical "miracle." Its lifesaving grinds along, three times weekly, month after month, with no end point or resolution—a very routine and tedious sort of wonder.

In the United States, at least, the success of extending care to all persons with renal failure has meant (as suggested earlier) that many recipients are too sick or old to conduct a fully active life. This equity of care has been attained through a unique federal program that highlights, through contrast, the inadequacies in the general provision of health care in the United States. The technical, organizational, and mercantile triumphs of commercial dialysis, and the invention and production of epoetin, would confirm to some Americans the advantages of free-market capitalism. Others, however, would question the huge profits derived from the care of persons with ESRD.

Perhaps "success" versus "failure" is the wrong way to assess maintenance dialysis. It can be looked upon as a complex set of interactions and debates involving sick people, doctors and nurses, government, and business. At 11:30 in the morning, a crampy patient and a nurse negotiate the last fifteen minutes "on the machine." Both, no doubt, would like to go home. Nephrologists at meetings and through our journals argue politely but endlessly about the relative importance of calcium versus phosphate in the well-being of persons with ESRD (some years after this book appears, the debates will turn to something else). The nephrology and dialysis "communities" in the United States repeatedly contend with Medicare over the latest attempts at cutbacks in reimbursement. Chronic hemodialysis has certainly become a "way of life" for more than the patients. Nurses, nephrologists, and Medicare functionaries tiring of all this can seek other work or maybe retire, but persons on dialysis can exit only through death or the treatment I have so far ignored—kidney transplantation, the subject of chapter 8.

CHAPTER EIGHT

The Gift of Life

A victim of renal failure, Alonzo "Zo" Mourning nonetheless returned to work in 2004. Ten months after receiving a kidney transplant, the star player in the National Basketball Association (NBA) and Olympic gold medalist was again landing shots and struggling against other giants for rebounds. His new kidney, formerly that of a generous cousin, enjoyed the protection of a specially designed padding: transplanted kidneys are placed into the lower abdomen and lack the protection that the rib cage provides "native" kidneys. "It's unbelievable," said a teammate with the New Jersey Nets. "This is a guy who almost died."[1] Mourning went on to play with much of his past vigor, even though at thirty-five he was already an old man by the standards of professional basketball, if a young one by standards of ESRD. As I write this in June of 2006, Zo—himself transplanted back to the Miami Heat, where he played before moving to the Nets—has just finished playing in the NBA championship finals. His time on the court was limited (in part owing to a recent muscle injury), but his team won. Mourning wanted to return to his job as a professional basketball player not because he needed the paychecks but because his work—which is to play—is what he loves, and at the time he had yet to play on a team that won the NBA championship.[2]

To return from renal failure to the NBA *at all* attests to Mourning's determination and his place within the sentimental-heroic tradition of great sports comebacks. As in the best of these stories, he overcame both grave illness and fear. To his credit, he more than once willingly expressed fear publicly. "Am I scared?" he said during a television interview in 2001, when he briefly returned to play while under treatment for his kidney disease (that is, before he reached the need for transplantation). "I'm extremely scared. I don't know what the future is going to bring."[3] His reappearance in the arena also proved the curative potential of transplantation. Kidney transplantation, though now a routine procedure, comes much closer to the mark as "medical miracle" than maintenance dialysis. Dialysis patients do not play in the NBA; they are more likely to watch it on their machine-side televisions.[4]

What led to the star athlete's transplantation? In 2000, a diagnosis of focal segmental glomerulosclerosis (FSGS) interrupted Mourning's career. His symptoms included those typical of Bright's Disease: dropsy (leg swelling), protein in the urine, and fatigue. As with most persons suffering with this particular form of glomerular disorder, he also showed worrisome elevation of his blood pressure. Despite receiving the most effective treatment known, in the form of pills by the handful, the brilliant player's disease progressed. Although he did return to play for a period while still on medication, it became clear that his future would bring either chronic dialysis or kidney transplantation. Most people with ESRD who receive a transplant have been on dialysis for some years awaiting a suitable "cadaver organ," a kidney made available from the body of someone who has died from something other than renal disease, very often from an accident or gunshot. But if someone alive is available to offer one of his or her kidneys, usually a relative, the person with failing kidneys can undergo "preemptive transplantation," that is, receive a new kidney before ever undergoing hemodialysis. Though medically desirable, preemptive transplantation requires optimal circumstances and coordination and remains an uncommon occurrence. Not surprisingly, even within a relatively equitable system, among Americans with ESRD preemptive transplantation tends to happen among those of higher socioeconomic status.

Alonzo Mourning was, of course, a wealthy professional athlete by the time his renal disease appeared. By custom, celebrities often become involved in some sort of advocacy or public awareness effort in relation to a disease, perhaps one known to the star's family, or, more rarely, to the star. Thus, in 2005, Mourning signed on to a program called "Rebound from Anemia," through which he would "visit U.S. clinics to educate about early warning signs."[5] Why "Rebound from *Anemia*" and not "from *Uremia*"? This program was sponsored by a pharmaceutical company, Ortho Biotech Products, which, in the complicated ways of its industry, became licensed to market Amgen's epoetin-alpha under a distinct trade name (Procrit) for the anemia of kidney failure in patients not yet on maintenance hemodialysis. "Take my advice," says Mourning in an Ortho Biotech press release, "if you're at risk for chronic kidney disease and have symptoms of anemia, speak to your doctor."[6] I do not assert that he received compensation from the company. Still, it is emblematically American for the star rebounder and transplant recipient in effect to endorse a star medication, recombinant epoetin, much as his teammates endorse brands of sneakers.

A 2005 press release from Ortho Biotech announcing "Rebound from Anemia" explains that those at risk for kidney disease include persons with diabetes or high blood pressure, those with a family history of such diseases, and "African-Americans, Hispanic-Americans, Asians, Pacific Islanders and American Indians." Alonzo Mourning, like many NBA stars, is African American, and so his story was covered in the popular African-American press. But the reader of the articles in *Jet* finds very little explicit portrayal of kidney disease as a particular affliction of blacks. "Blacks, especially males, are hard hit by kidney disease due to the high rate of high blood pressure and diabetes," amounts to the entire discussion of this important association within several articles in *Jet* about Mourning and about Sean Elliott, another black NBA player who had FSGS.[7]

As I suggested in chapter 7, this linkage of a disease with an ethnic group raises abundant cautionary flags and difficulties, as fully explored in historian Keith Wailoo's writings on sickle-cell anemia.[8] Suffice it to repeat here that African Americans can do without the stigma of being known for "weak" or disease-prone kidneys. Yet, during the last quarter of the twentieth century and the early years of the twenty-first, plentiful evidence has shown that early detection and adequate treatment of hypertension and proteinuria with medication *can* lessen the risk of some renal diseases reaching end stage. Prevention rarely makes headlines. Alonzo Mourning's remarkable story tells rather of a celebrity growing more heroic when his mysterious and unpronounceable kidney disease was defeated by a celebrity among operations—major organ transplantation. As previously stated, one encounters a quiet and enduring heroism in the lives of countless dialysis recipients trying to live as full lives as they can. With successful transplantation, however, the valor occurs during a transformative and victorious few hours, in another arena of vanquishers, the modern operating room.

BEGINNINGS OF KIDNEY TRANSPLANTATION

It is remarkable that the kidney happened to be the first internal organ subject to replacement both by a machine and by an actual substitute from another person.[9] Each human kidney connects to the body usually by way of one artery, one vein, and a ureter that drains urine into the bladder. Thus the surgical obstacles seemed relatively few, and indeed the first experimental implantations of kidneys in animals carried out in the early twentieth century were linked to the invention of techniques for joining (or "anastomosing") blood vessels. Most widely known among those pursuing such work, the French, and later American, surgeon and researcher Alexis Carrel (1873–1944) received a Nobel Prize in 1912, indicating the prompt and extraordinary attention given to surgical transplantation. Prior to the 1940s, a few scattered and now obscure surgeons attempted the transplantation of human or animal kidneys into persons near death with renal failure. They are obscure because their precocious attempts did not turn out very well, and in some cases because they toiled outside the mainstream of Western medicine. One such individual, U. U. (or Yu Yu) Voronoy, performed six renal transplants in Russia beginning in 1936 and published his accounts in Russian and Spanish medical journals. His first patient was a young woman with acute renal failure from ingestion of corrosive sublimate (mercuric chloride), the same toxic substance encountered in chapter 5 in the story of

E.R., the young woman given dialysis treatment at Mount Sinai Hospital in 1948.

At about the same time, in 1947, several surgeons at Boston's Peter Bent Brigham Hospital in conjunction with internist and renal authority George Thorn performed a human kidney transplantation on a young woman. They had been carrying out experimental studies of organ transplantation in dogs. Recall that Thorn made his hospital one of the first centers for development of the artificial kidney (chapter 5). In some earlier accounts, the woman who received the kidney (sewn into blood vessels of her upper arm) was described as having suffered acute renal failure from "an infection of the uterus," bleeding, and shock, while pregnant. The "coded" understanding would be that the inciting event was an abortion gone wrong.[10] The group of young physicians and surgeons hoped that if the transplanted kidney (obtained, with family permission, from a patient near death) could function even briefly, time might be won for the woman's kidneys to regain function. The idea was the same as using an artificial kidney in a similar situation. The grafted kidney worked for several days, and in fact the woman's own kidneys did recover, and she survived this illness.[11] There was no way to know if she might have done so without the more or less improvised transplantation, but the event stimulated further interest in both transplantation and dialysis, at least at the Brigham.

Thorn, who died in 2004 at the age of ninety-eight, maintained an astonishing vigor and capacious memory almost until his last days. In 1991, I had the privilege of interviewing Dr. Thorn as part of an oral history project of the Harvard Medical School. At that time, he had come to remember the patient as a young woman "who had had a baby and had a terrible hemorrhage afterwards and had gone into shock . . . so that her kidneys shut down." He also recalled that the "woman lived and her baby lived." I don't know which account is true: in an 1981 memoir, Thorn had referred to the patient's "uterine infection and blood loss."[12] The 1947 transplantation became a hallmark in Thorn's reflection on his career and on the orderly story of advance in renal care at his hospital, as he knew it. Perhaps even his robust memory eventually permitted reshaping of the narrative—to a more pure and perfect representation of worthy benefits won through daring and progress in medicine. Nonetheless, there remains an undeniable linkage of the origins of "renal replacement therapy" with illegal abortions gone wrong.

In 1950, a surgeon in Chicago named Richard Lawler transplanted a kidney from a person who had died from liver failure into a woman uremic from polycystic kidney disease, an inherited disorder. The transplanted kidney functioned for at least several months, but the woman lived for five more years, presumably from some unexpected recovery of filtration by her own diseased kidneys. Over the next few years, transplantation was attempted by French surgeons and clinicians Charles Dubost, Marcel Servelle, René Küss, Jean Hamburger, and others. Dubost and Servelle obtained their kidneys (with official sanction) from a guillotined convict, adding another somewhat sordid element to the pioneering years of organ transplantation.[13] In Toronto, the individualistic surgeon Gordon Murray, also an inventor of an artificial kidney, carried out four transplants in the early 1950s. Only the fourth met with success, as a woman with advanced Bright's Disease and severe edema displayed an impressive diuresis and recovery of health: "Transplanted Kidney Saves Dying Woman" headlined a Toronto newspaper. She lived for many years, but skeptics suspected that her own kidneys had somehow recovered, and Murray did no follow-up testing.[14] In Boston, surgeon David Hume at the Peter Bent Brigham Hospital, in conjunction with John P. Merrill and George Thorn, carried out a series of transplants into persons with chronic renal failure from 1951 to 1953. They were able to first improve the medical status of the recipients through use of their rotating-drum artificial kidney. Several of these grafted kidneys did function for a matter of months, but none longer. The group concluded that "at the present state of our knowledge, renal homotransplants do not appear to be justified in the treatment of human disease."[15]

By this time, numerous observations in experimental biology had made it clear that an animal or human being usually reacts to cells or tissue transplanted from another individual as foreign, or "nonself." The engrafted material would be destroyed by a response that came to be known as immunological rejection.

Much of the foundation for this understanding came from extensive studies of skin grafting by British biologist Peter Medawar
(1915–1987) and his co-workers; Medawar with Macfarlane Burnet
received the Nobel Prize for Physiology or Medicine in 1960. The
general lack of success with human kidney transplantation in the
early 1950s, despite adequate surgical techniques, seemed to confirm that "rejection" was at fault. Efforts then focused on finding
ways to reduce the body's normal immunological activity so that
the foreign kidney might be tolerated. This, of course, is a dicey
sort of business, since the same set of responses allows the body
to defend itself from a huge range of potentially dangerous bacteria and other microbes and also plays a role in the suppression
of some cancer cells. Nonetheless, with the hope of prolonging
the lives of people with terminal kidney disease, and in the period
before the availability of long-term dialysis, the early transplanters tried irradiation to the body, or cortisone, to partly defeat the
immune response.

Amidst these discouraging attempts, chance offered a remarkable opportunity to the Brigham physicians and surgeons. In 1954,
a twenty-four-year-old man in Boston with failing kidneys from
Bright's Disease (or glomerulonephritis) and severe high blood
pressure was known to have a healthy identical twin brother. The
man's astute physician (a Dr. David C. Miller of the U.S. Public
Health Service) knew of the transplantation work at the Brigham
Hospital. Dr. Miller also apparently understood that rejection
ought not to occur between identical twins, who would share
their entire "antigenic" makeup. Joseph E. Murray (b. 1919) had
replaced David Hume as the surgical head of the renal team at the
Brigham, which agreed to consider the possibility. Organ donation has always raised ethical questions, and the man's twin was
appraised of the known risks. It was understood long before 1954
that a healthy person can live entirely normally with one kidney.
When an otherwise well person loses one kidney (e.g., as a donor,
or from trauma), the remaining kidney soon "hypertrophies" to
increase (though not fully double) its filtering capacity. Still, the
outcome of the unprecedented procedure was uncertain at best,
and surgery always brings risk. In addition, although glomerulonephritis is not typically a familial disease, it was pertinent to

consider the threat of the same or similar ailment occurring in the donating brother. Many persons, including physicians, still saw most chronic diseases as "running in families," a continuation of pervasive hereditarian ideas from the nineteenth century. Of course, some chronic diseases indeed do show a familial pattern.

The transfer of a kidney from one twin to the other on December 23, 1954, met with success. Richard Herrick, the recipient, went back to work, married a nurse, and became a father. Regrettably, he died eight years after the transplant of a heart attack, probably a complication of the hypertension and blood lipid alterations that occur with the long-standing proteinuric renal disease that led to the transplantation.[16] The first kidney transplantation between identical twins attracted immense coverage by the media, somewhat to the discomfort of Murray and the medical leader of renal work at the Brigham, John Merrill. The borrowing of organs was, of course, itself novel and exotic, and a kind of mystery and strangeness has always surrounded identical twins. It is no doubt very odd to go through life with a perfect double, even without the occasion for one's double to serve as a spare parts shelf. Amazingly, Murray and the Boston group carried out six more renal transplants in identical twins, and others soon took place elsewhere in North America and Europe. Though this strategy obviously could not help very many of those reaching terminal kidney failure, the successes proved the technical feasibility of renal transplantation and showed that a kidney could function well without its nerve supply (no attempt is made to restore it, and this was an unknown).

The reappearance of proteinuria in some of the recipient twins after several years did alarm and disappoint, even if the overall kidney function stayed adequate. The physicians interpreted the proteinuria as recurrence of the previous glomerulonephritis in the new kidney. Later information confirmed that indeed some glomerular kidney diseases *do* recur in the transplanted organ. This finding helped shed light on the mechanism, already supposed to be somehow immunologic, of most of these proteinuric disorders that together once formed "Bright's Disease." The lesson was that the "disease" has to be in part something present in the bloodstream or entire body, not just the kidney. Richard Bright had suspected that this was the case in his Guy's patients of the 1820s and 1830s—some sort of "inflammatory" state of the whole system. The ideas of humoralism, and of "sympathy," which were his inheritance to use and expand, favored an admixture of local and systemic understandings. But we are well beyond Bright and need to move along.

THE MATURITY OF KIDNEY TRANSPLANTATION

Obviously, transplantation between identical twins could not help very many persons with kidney failure. But these successes prompted the Boston group and Jean Hamburger's team in Paris to carry out transplants between fraternal (dizygotic) twins, using steroids and radiation to combat rejection. In France, René Küss performed the first renal transplantation between nontwin siblings in 1960, using irradiation as the immunosuppressant. He then attempted transplants between nonsiblings, adding steroids and the new drug 6-mercaptopurine. It was Roy Calne in London who began experimental work with this promising drug, which reduced proliferation of certain white cells that contribute to the immune attack on grafts, but it proved difficult to dose safely. Working at the Peter Bent Brigham Hospital in Boston with the Murray-Merrill group, Calne did transplants in dogs to study the use of a closely related drug, azathioprine, which proved much easier to use. For the next twenty years, the combination of steroids (cortisone-like drugs, mainly prednisone) and azathioprine served as the primary means of achieving partial immunosuppression for renal transplantation. It allowed transplanters in North America and France to achieve graft survival of a year or more using "cadaver kidneys," harvested from persons recently deceased. Thus, renal transplantation fostered acceptance of the concept of brain death, or the "heart-beating cadaver," from whom—with appropriate family consent—organs could be removed before suffering irreparable injury from lack of blood flow. Kidney disease, long feared as a pathway to death, came to help redefine death.

Also in the 1960s, laboratory researchers devised the process of "tissue typing" to obtain the optimal match of recipient to a cadaver kidney (this inelegant phrase became standard usage, though it has been replaced by the more delicate "deceased donor kidney"). Analogous to the red blood cell types, which are matched for blood transfusion, other cells of the body carry inherited protein markers, or antigens, though this system is more complex. Maximizing the number of antigenic matches can lessen the chances that the recipient's immune system will destroy a transplanted organ (some immunosuppression will still be required). As renal transplantation spread from a few research centers to many hospitals, the intent to achieve the best antigen match gave rise to a national system for doing so in the United States (and similarly elsewhere) as once again technologies meshed.

Machines to cool and preserve recently harvested kidneys and the widespread availability of air travel allowed the organs to be moved as necessary from one region to another. Thus, if a set of kidneys became available following a fatal auto accident in, say, Chicago, they might be flown to Cleveland and Memphis to seek the most favorable matches, bypassing dialysis patients on the waiting lists in Illinois. One might try to imagine these iced and isolated kidneys flying through the skies, precious passengers whose immunologic identities can trump the pleas and hopes of prospective recipients on the ground far below, tethered to their hemodialysis machines. I have related in earlier chapters that dropsy and Bright's Disease counted among those chronic maladies that medicine believed could be cured by *travel*. Now, oddly, healthy kidneys, risen from dead bodies and for a time out on their own in the world, were doing the travel, in search of latter-day patients. Some of the recipients did journey as well to meet their kidneys at a regional transplant center. This organ-sharing process required considerable organization and efficiency, but unlike the situation with chronic hemodialysis, no commercial system emerged. The nonprofit organization that does this work in the United States is called UNOS, the United Network for Organ Sharing. The matching plan grew in sophistication as transplant surgeons and other parties eventually agreed upon a "point" system to balance the gains of optimal matching against the number of years a particular individual had been waiting for a kidney. This modification in part addressed the troubling awareness that blacks on dialysis for a variety of reasons tended to wait longer for transplantation.[17]

In the late 1970s, it was again the distinguished British transplant surgeon and scientist Roy Calne leading the way with the
introduction of the drug cyclosporin, representing a new class of
agents called calcineurin inhibitors. Cyclosporin (and the later
drug of the same type, tacrolimus) inhibits the activity of a segment of the immune system whose functions include the rejection of grafts, but it does not suppress all bodily defenses. It was
the most effective transplant drug so far developed, a verifiable
"breakthrough."[18] The new agent, used in conjunction with steroids, moved one-year transplant survival into the unprecedented
90 percent range. The power of cyclosporin to block rejection
made tissue typing and matching less essential and greatly expanded the possibilities for renal transplantation.

Other new methods of focused immunosuppression introduced in the 1980s and 1990s, as well as improved surgical techniques, also played a role. Living donors no longer needed to be
blood relatives: spouses and friends could now offer a kidney with
reasonable confidence that the extraordinary gift would succeed in
bettering the life of the recipient. Cyclosporin's effectiveness (and
the other advances) led to new, sometimes agonizing, ethical and
emotional deliberations. How much obligation should a spouse
or relative feel to donate a kidney? Should someone with ESRD
accept the tendering of a kidney from a co-worker or relatively ca-
sual friend—and what, if not altruism, might sometimes underlie
such an offer? Anthropologists teach that gift-giving implies exchange in most cultures: what, if any, obligations accompany the
acceptance of the gift of a body part? The number of organs (kidneys and others) available for transplantation falls far short of the
demand: how much should the medical profession, allied health
advocacy organizations, and government press the public to think
about donation or even provide incentives? What are the potential
conflicts of interest for physicians? And, finally, what is no doubt
the most provocative of the new questions: should body parts be
sold?[19]

Transplantation statistics for 2003 in the United States (the
most recent available as I write this) show that about 128,000 persons were living with a functioning kidney graft, and about 16,000
transplantations had been performed.[20] A simple international

compilation is not available, but many thousands are done each year throughout the world. Other figures for the United States show that the chance of a deceased donor kidney working adequately one year after transplantation is 89 percent, and 67 percent at five years. For a living donor kidney, the numbers are 95 percent and 80 percent.[21] These results would have been much envied twenty years earlier, and most practitioners of nephrology now consider transplantation the preferred treatment of ESRD, even with its hazards and emotional demands.

THE EXPERIENCE AND MORAL MEANINGS OF TRANSPLANTATION

I have already presented the story of Alonzo Mourning, whose new kidney returned him to professional basketball and his first championship season. Unlike Mr. Mourning, most people with ESRD who receive a transplant have been on dialysis for at least months, and often years, awaiting a deceased donor organ. Others, like Mourning, do benefit from the generosity of a relative or friend and can plan the transplantation to occur when mild uremic symptoms first appear. But for persons who have become ill from their renal failure, then passed some time on dialysis, transplantation—when it works—can indeed be transformative, virtually a "cure." Patients who endured complications of hemodialysis or simply never felt well with it can feel fine again, while those whom the machine kept mostly without symptoms regain the sense and reality of freedom. "I felt good again. I had my appetite, my energy," a transplant recipient in Rochester, New York, told a news reporter. "Before my transplant," another recounted for a protransplant Web site, "there were days when I would come home from dialysis and I couldn't even walk up my front steps. . . . Now I can do anything—absolutely anything." For another person on dialysis, most striking was liberation from that torment of the renal patient, restriction of fluid intake: "Suddenly, for the first time in years, I was drinking as much as I wanted. I turned in my thimble for a stein and made good and frequent use of it."[22]

Renal transplantation, though wondrous when all goes well, can, however, provide its own anxieties, complications, and even—though very rarely—the possibility of sudden demise on the operating table. Years may pass for someone on the transplant waiting list, hoping not to be spending a weekend away, or even at the movies, when the phone call might come. Here, again, new technologies almost playfully find their alliances—that patient in the 1980s obtained a pager, now it's a mobile phone. Of course, gratitude mixes with worry when a loved one offers a kidney, and sometimes remorse and guilt supervene if the transplant fails. The first days and week after the operation have been termed "nerve-wracking" by many recipients. Occasionally, a cadaver kidney has suffered some injury from its period without normal blood flow; then, its new owner and the transplant team wait in agony for it to "open up." Though less commonly encountered now than in the earlier years of renal transplantation, acute rejection remains a risk. It can usually be reversed with treatment, but patients and transplant team suffer nervously through the setback. Although a transplanted kidney may function adequately for decades, most gradually lose activity from a complex of processes referred to as chronic rejection or more recently as chronic allograft nephropathy. The transplanted kidney begins to leak protein into the urine, and blood creatinine slowly rises, as filtering power lessens: the "new" kidney in effect acquires its own new case of Bright's Disease.

I earlier referred to the person receiving dialysis for ESRD as a new type of patient, a "specialist" among the chronically ill, in effect carrying out a complex job. In fact, ESRD can evolve into a career, or at least something like a long series of promotions and demotions within a turbulent sort of company. It has not been unusual for someone to receive hemodialysis for half a decade or more, then receive a cadaver transplant that works for some years but fades out. Second and even third attempts are common. The following story is not out of the ordinary: A young woman lost her kidney function owing to the disease lupus erythematosus at the age of sixteen. After six months on dialysis her mother gave her a kidney, which rejected after two years. Back she went to hemodialysis during her college years and her twenties. A second kidney transplant "ended the day after I received it due to a blood clot." Eventually a third transplant proved successful: she no longer had to "rely on a machine that I hated." Five years later, now a school teacher with a master's degree, she and her third donated kidney were doing well.[23]

Even when chronic allograft nephropathy claims a transplanted kidney, it may have kept its recipient productive and feeling well for five, ten, or more years. But there are some other risks, particularly from the immunosuppressive drugs. Cyclosporin, which so much advanced the ability to transplant, ironically can itself cause toxicity to the kidneys and lead to some other side effect. Steroids, usually in the form of tablets of prednisone, can produce a range of side effects, including weight gain, high blood sugar, changes in the skin, and cataracts of the eyes. By virtue of what they do, the immunosuppressive drugs of course make the transplanted individual vulnerable to infections. Whereas bacterial urinary infections are very common and easily treated, persons taking agents that reduce the body's immune responses raise susceptibility to rare microbial diseases such as cytomegalovirus infection, pneumonia from pneumocystis, and polyoma virus. The latter virus attacks the transplanted kidney, often resulting in its loss. Finally, the immunosuppression puts the recipient at risk for certain cancers, particularly of the skin and lymphatic system (lymphomas). Oddly, otherwise common cancers of the colon, breast, or lung do not occur with increased frequency. Although the risk of a life-threatening infection or malignancy is small, some patients read the warnings and choose to stay with dialysis if they have been managing to get along with it and its obligations.

Although donors rarely suffer any serious complications, their experience cannot be looked upon as trifling. Even with modern laparoscopic methods that reduce surgical invasiveness, the organ-harvesting operation requires general anesthesia and considerable cutting through the body wall. Postoperative pain and sometimes nausea can be considerable. Many persons require several weeks or months before feeling entirely robust after any sort of major operation or exposure to general anesthetic. Whereas successful renal transplantation moves the recipient from the world of the sick to that of the well, for the donor it forces a sudden travel in the opposite direction, though the visit is temporary.[24]

In chapter 7, I referred to a pamphlet comprising mainly photographs published by the U.S. Public Health Service in 1968, titled *A Chance to Live.* At the time, the service was supporting several pilot chronic dialysis units. The pamphlet conveys a decidedly optimistic viewpoint, especially the section called "Family Man," and calls the artificial kidney a "miracle of modern medical technology."[25] But it also refers to the "difficulties, frustrations, inconveniences, and tensions" associated with chronic dialysis. No one then even knew about dialysis-associated bone disease, amyloid deposits in joints, and some of the other long-term problems. A segment about a teenage boy, "Looking Ahead," speaks to the uncertainty of his future and states that transplantation, not his current artificial kidney, offers him the best hope for a normal life. I have no idea who in the Kidney Disease Control Program of the U.S. Public Health Service chose the title, *A Chance to Live,* or with how much deliberation. In a sense, the title suggests that in 1968 at least, dialysis did not seem to promise much—a "chance" . . . and merely "to live." True, this is no small thing for someone facing death from organ failure.

But transplantation offers the *gift of life.* Through the wondrous technology of computer-based searching, one can readily find countless stories of transplantation—kidney, heart, liver, pancreas, and so on—in newspapers, magazines, and of course Web sites. The published stories of renal transplantation have these sorts of titles (many titles are used several times): "A Mother's Gift," "The Gift that Saved My Life," "Living because Someone Else Had Died," "A Teacher's Gift? Why, Most Certainly," "A Brother's Love: When Crisis Hits Home," "The True Meaning of 'Brotherly Love,'" "Transplant: Saving a Life Is a Mitzvah," "A Father's Day Story: A Son's Sacrifice for His Best Friend," "A Stranger's Surprise Gift," and "The Gift of Life."[26]

These sentimental headings introduce remarkable stories of courage and deep generosity. A forty-two-year-old white middle-school teacher in Fayetteville, North Carolina, offered a kidney to one of her students, a fourteen-year-old African-American boy. "I instantly knew that this was something I could do," she told a *New York Times* reporter. "In this world, you need to realize that there's a bond. There's a connection between you and everybody else you see." The youth's mother concluded that "God chose us together to accomplish his purpose."[27] Said a donating brother in

San Bernardino, California: "There was never a question. . . . I had two kidneys and had never been sick. . . . You could say God just took control. . . . I'm still Larry, he's still Carl, and we're still brothers, and no difference."[28] Another brother of a man with ESRD, in Cleveland, Ohio, stated: "Because he is my brother, to me there is no matter of a decision, there is no reason for deep thought." He added in his interview with a reporter that "if God has a hand in it, everything will be alright."[29] A woman in London, England, told her best friend with worsening kidney function that "I've got two kidneys, I don't need both so you can have one." The "stunned" friend started crying. Later, recovered and feeling "normal again" after attending a concert, she wept again: "Alex has given me my life back."[30]

Finally, we have "Sharing More Than a Corner of the Office," a story *about* reporters. Three "pod mates" in the financial news staff of the *Washington Post* had over many years become close friends. One of them, Warren Brown, was doing poorly on dialysis after a transplanted kidney from his wife had failed. His friend and colleague Martha McNeil Hamilton observed this and offered one of her kidneys. According to the writer summarizing the reporters' story, "for Brown, the fact that it's Hamilton's kidney and not a stranger's makes a big difference." The recipient, recovering after an unusually complicated operation and postoperative course, explained this notion: "It's not just a matter of transplanting an organ. As silly as it may sound, I truly believe that you accept something of [that] person's spirit."[31] I had never before encountered the idea of kidney as something like habitat of soul, but sensibilities similar to that expressed by Warren Brown are known to be common among donors (or their families) and recipients of transplanted organs, particularly, of course, hearts.[32] Transplant surgeons tend to view such animistic beliefs with skepticism, if not as outright creepy. The author of the story about the *Washington Post* colleagues did not mention (though it's evident from accompanying photographs) that the donor was white, and the recipient yet another black sufferer of kidney disease. Recipients of deceased donor kidneys may also, of course, know feelings of gratitude and grace. Said a transplant recipient in Sacramento, California, who might speak for tens of thousands, "For the rest of my life, I will appreciate and be thankful that my donor and his/her family had the compassion and love to do this for me."[33]

These transplant stories, as I have noted, abound in the popular press and on the Internet. They rarely hail the accomplishments of applied medical immunology, the technology of organ pres-ervation, or even the surgeon's hand and (recently) laparoscope. Names of surgeons or nephrologists appear infrequently, and one does not read praise for cyclosporin. These narratives tell instead of gift-giving, love, and above all, human relationships—bonds between siblings, parent and child, teacher and pupil, old friends, even between the living and the dead. The writers and editors know their business, and what will grip readers. The campaigns to encourage organ donation instruct the public that human gen-erosity and the belief that one person should help another make possible the "miracle" of organ transplantation. But the converse can claim truth as well: organ transplantation has made possible an unprecedented form and depth of generosity, something new within human interaction—what a philosopher named Hans Jo-nas termed a gift "beyond duty and claim."[34]

These thousands of instances of gift-giving and connection have generated a community of transplant recipients, donor families, and living donors, which gathers at extraordinary events known as the U.S. Transplant Games and World Transplant Games.[35] The U.S. Games were first held in Texas in 1982 and only a few partici-pants attended. By the year 2000, over 7,000 recipients, donors, donor families, professionals, and friends appeared to compete as regional teams in a wide range of sports, as well as to participate in ceremonies, social events, and educational activities. The National Donor Recognition Ceremony, initiated in 1998, provides an op-portunity for recipients and workers in the field to demonstrate their gratitude. It is a powerful moment when the donor families and living donors proceed into the arena at the opening ceremo-nies, met by the standing ovation of the gathered recipients, fami-lies, and friends. The U.S. Transplant Games, sponsored by the National Kidney Foundation, are of course a media event that serves to call attention to the need for organ donation. Not sur-prisingly, pharmaceutical companies that manufacture the promi-nent immunosuppressive agents have supported the games as a public service. The World Transplant Games (formerly the Transplant Olympics) are organized by the World Transplant Games Federation and held in odd-numbered years.

It is obvious also from the small number of stories sampled above that those persons participating in the powerful experience of kidney transplantation may situate the event as well within the connections between human beings and God. This is so at least in the United States, where the nurturing of state-church separation belies a historically pervasive Christian framework, the theology of which rests on themes of sacrifice and exalted gift-giving.[36] Certainly patients expressing their feelings about dialysis have also offered thanks to the Divine, but this seems to occur more regularly and powerfully with transplantation. Recipients (Christian or otherwise) sometimes know a feeling of salvation and look upon the transplantation itself and the act of the donation as blessed.

Mythic stories dealing with the transfer or giving of body parts—eyes, legs, hearts—are found in ancient literature of both Asia and the West.[37] In the early twenty-first century, transplantation of the kidney, heart, lung, and other organs, though a still imperfect practice, can be carried out with relative safety and, at least for kidneys, a high probability of restored well-being for many years. Transplantation counts as an unequivocal success story of the modern operating room and affirms the virtues of high-technology medicine. Within American society—which seems afflicted with incivility, violence, and racism—the act of donation exemplifies as well a different sort of virtue—altruism and human connection. Beyond even this, some recipients of a kidney transplant can see in the returning trickle of urine the very presence of a loving God.

CHAPTER NINE

Progression
and Renewal

—◦◦◦—

Basketball star Alonzo Mourning stood among those who experienced their kidney transplantation in a religious context. "I was just giving praise and thanks," he explained in one postgame interview: he had "pointed to the sky" after hitting his first posttransplant shot (a 15-footer). "Jason was definitely God-sent," Mourning had earlier said of his cousin and donor. "I'm very grateful."[1] Whereas this world-class athlete voiced his gratitude to God, his cousin, and probably somewhere else to his nurses, physicians, and transplant surgeon, he would have had reason to wonder why the hand of medicine, whether guided by science or deity, could neither prevent nor cure his original kidney-destroying disease.

PRELUDE TO PREVENTION

Readers may recall that focal segmental glomerulosclerosis (FSGS), discussed briefly in earlier chapters, was as one of the forms of proteinuric kidney disease defined by renal biopsy. FSGS is a disease of the glomeruli, the critical sieve-like microscopic tufts of blood capillaries that filter out bodily wastes, while retaining essential substances, as they make the fluid that will become urine. FSGS leads to massive proteinuria and the consequent renal salt and water retention that becomes edema. If this particular disorder existed in earlier times—and there is no reason to doubt that it did—it would have been understood as dropsy, then later as

Bright's Disease, and now, as one cause of the nephrotic syndrome and kidney failure.[2] Current classification sees it as comprising five subtypes, the "tip variant," "perihilar variant," "collapsing form," and so on. Once comparatively rare, since the 1990s FSGS has been showing up at alarming rates, and it is particularly common among blacks. Of course, this malady has attracted research and funding. A "circulating factor" that seems to induce the glomerular "leakiness" for protein has been identified in the blood of some persons with FSGS. An enormous amount of investigation since the 1980s has revealed that the filtering, or "sieving," structure is almost incomprehensibly complex at the molecular level. It consists of numerous structural elements with newly fashioned names like "nephrin" and "podocin" forming a system of latticeworks and pores. The genes for most of these structural proteins are known, and mutations in some of them will cause proteinuria, though very few people suffer from a clear-cut inherited form of the disease.[3]

In fact, there exists a profound gap between the accumulation of descriptive knowledge of FSGS and any real understanding of it. No one can assemble the mass of observations into any coherent story, at least as I write this. No one knows its cause or why it occurs more frequently in persons of color.[4] It is treated with high doses of steroids (cortisone-like drugs), but not every patient responds, and many sustain one or more side effects of the drug. In a sense, and the sense that matters to patients, as of the first decade of the twenty-first century we understand this form of Bright's Disease no better than Bright understood the cases he treated in nineteenth-century London. Actually, Bright was *better* able to formulate a plausible explanation of proteinuric renal disease in the 1830s, in the context of medical theory then, than nephrologists can do for much of it now—whatever we may think of "sympathy" and the "suppression of insensible perspiration" (see chapter 3). Alonzo Mourning received the best possible care guided by a nephrologist with unsurpassed expertise and experience in glomerular disorders, but still his kidneys plummeted to end stage within a few years of diagnosis. And since so little is known about the cause or basis of FSGS, if Mr. Mourning had asked his nephrologist what his family, friends, teammates, or even fans might do to prevent its onset in one of them, no good answer would have been available.

As discussed in earlier chapters, far exceeding FSGS as a cause of ESRD is diabetes, particularly the so-called type 2, previously known as "adult-onset." Certainly not all persons with diabetes incur renal disease: probably some genetic predisposition also plays a role. For type 2 diabetes, something is known about prevention—regular exercise and avoiding obesity can reduce its likelihood, even among persons with a family history. But, at least in the United States of the early twenty-first century, obesity abounds and too few exercise, so diabetes attains "epidemic" proportions, in turn producing numerous cases of kidney failure.

And so it is possible to suggest, looking back, that there has been a "disconnect" in the science and care of renal disease during the mid- and late twentieth century. In the United States, technologically and organizationally effective means arose to treat hundreds of thousands of cases of kidney failure with dialysis or transplantation, while comparatively little was learned about preventing the disease. A search of the National Library of Medicine's Medline database of published medical articles reveals that from 1975 through 1985, when dialysis centers proliferated, only forty-eight articles were indexed as dealing with prevention of chronic kidney failure. Scanning the titles suggests that many of these were only marginally about prevention and that others dealt with what would be called secondary or tertiary prevention—that is, not preventing a disease as such, but avoiding recurrences or complications once it is present. Maybe prevention presents a more difficult problem than building artificial organs, especially since there is not just one type of chronic, progressive kidney disease. But likely other factors played a role. Physicians feel an imperative to find some treatment for a serious disease presented to them, and dialysis or transplantation offered this for kidney failure.

Also, generally speaking, prevention simply does not attract the interest or attention of physicians nearly as much as do diagnosis, treatment, and—for academicians—exploration of underlying mechanisms of disease. Preventive medicine typically occupies a marginal place and status within American medical schools. It is nonetheless the case that the great gains in life expectancy and well-being of humankind over the last two hundred years have resulted from preventive measures—for example, improvement in water supplies, eradication of disease-carrying mosquitoes, and immunizations.

Nephrology in the United States offers an illustration of priorities.[5] It formed in the 1950s and 1960s, comprising mainly research physicians and scientists at medical schools interested in the physiology of the kidney, and a smaller contingent devoted to dialysis and the treatment of renal failure. The physiologist-nephrologists particularly favored elegant studies of the normal function of the kidney tubule; this was referred to as "transport"—the movement of substances from inside the tubule, across its cellular wall, and into the surrounding capillary blood. They had inherited from earlier periods a model of kidney function that saw the glomerulus as a simple mechanical filter and the tubule as the more subtle and adaptive component of the nephron unit. The tubule seemed to be the thinking part of the kidney, and these doctors were curious, thinking men.[6] Some of the researchers worked at the National Institutes of Health, which through its expanding program of "extramural" grants also paid for much of the laboratory work at medical schools. The policy of the NIH at that time created "a medical research program of scientists by scientists." Researchers would enjoy complete freedom to choose their projects without concern for obvious clinical usefulness.[7] We have seen in previous chapters that early dialysis units received funding from the U.S. Public Health Service (of which NIH is a major component); then Medicare established the ESRD reimbursement program (dialysis and transplantation). Though some nephrologists in the United States, and certainly elsewhere, did choose to study the causes and foundations of kidney disease itself, through the 1970s and into the 1980s, the American government was paying mostly for the care of persons with end-stage disease, and for esoteric investigations of tubular "transport," to be reported in the *American Journal of Physiology.*

A NEW HOPE: HYPERFILTRATION AND THE KEY TO PROGRESSION

Then, in the early 1980s, a new direction for the future of kidney disease in the United States, and eventually the world, emerged. Some nephrologists looked around with alarm at the swelling number of persons enrolling for dialysis or transplants, and a few looked backward, to the work and ideas of earlier students of kidney disease, such as Thomas Addis. He and other physicians interested in renal ailments in the 1930s knew that no artificial kidney or transplantation existed to aid chronic patients whose course ran downhill, so they sought to preserve renal viability through diet. In 1982, nephrologist Barry Brenner, of Harvard Medical School and the Peter Bent Brigham Hospital in Boston, with his colleagues, published a review article in the prestigious (and also Boston-based) *New England Journal of Medicine* that called attention to a potential means of preventing or at least delaying ESRD.[8] They did so by offering a concept for understanding the seemingly inevitable deterioration of kidneys once serious renal disease has appeared. Brenner had trained and worked in the laboratories of the NIH, and like others in the late 1960s used a technique called micropuncture to uncover the mechanisms of tubular transport. Brenner, however, using a suitable strain of rat for the purpose, eventually turned his attention to the glomerulus, the primary filtering structure, largely ignored by researchers though it was known to be the seat of many renal diseases in humans. A voracious reader, Brenner also knew something of the history of treating renal disease before the period of dialysis, including the largely forgotten ideas of Addis, which were cited in the first sentence of that landmark 1982 article.

Brenner's laboratory showed in rats that when most nephrons were destroyed, remaining glomeruli adapted to increase their contribution to filtration by elevating pressure in the structure.[9] This elevated pressure, though perhaps providing a short-term benefit, Brenner suggested, eventually caused the remaining glomeruli to suffer a kind of wear-and-tear injury, as might remaining cylinders and pistons in an eight-cylinder engine with three or four cylinders out of commission. Since protein ingestion itself tends to maximize renal filtration, the low-protein diet might ease the overwork of remaining nephrons, thus slowing the spiral of more and more loss of working units. This was, to some extent, a reformulation of Thomas Addis's concept, with "hyperfiltration" taking the place of "work."

Brenner's team was not alone in thinking and working along these lines: Tetsuo Shimamura and Ashton B. Morrison at Rutgers Medical School in New Jersey were doing so, as were MacKenzie Walser and colleagues at Johns Hopkins University.[10] Also in the 1980s, researchers in Europe displayed convincing evidence that among persons with both diabetes and hypertension, effective lowering of the blood pressure with medication slowed the worsening of diabetic renal disease—presumably high blood pressure in the body as a whole led to high pressure in glomeruli.[11] But Barry Brenner and his group more persuasively than the others propelled the hyperfiltration hypothesis forward because: they demonstrated the actual phenomenon using the nephrologist's most honored laboratory technique, micropuncture; constructed an encompassing framework that included a treatment outcome (the resurrected low-protein diet); enjoyed the imprimatur of the Harvard Medical School; and published a lucid overview of their findings and ideas in the *New England Journal of Medicine,* a periodical of scriptural standing in the world of medicine.

Before long, wherever nephrologists gathered, the words "hyperfiltration" and "progression" were to be heard, as well as calls to nutritionists to teach the low-protein diet to patients with chronic renal disease. (Recalling the singular experience of Tom Addis and Ava Helen Pauling treating Linus Pauling's renal disease—from chapter 4—most of the dieticians enlisted to play a central role were women.) "Progression" referred to progress *downward* in renal function, marked by the gradual up-creeping of the blood creatinine measurement, the standard indicator of renal filtration capacity. That the low-protein diet and better control of blood pressure might slow this progression both encouraged and fascinated nephrologists, even those whose income depended in good part on full shifts in the dialysis unit. Everyone knew, however, that persons with early forms of renal disease, who generally still felt well, would have a hard time maintaining a low-protein diet, especially in hamburger-rich America. Furthermore, no large clinical trial had proved its worth in a sizeable population of patients; and an overly zealous, or unskilled, enforcement of protein restriction risked a form of malnutrition.

Thus, prominent nephrologists, shapers of opinion, came to sort themselves out as enthusiasts or skeptics (and of course some merely reserved judgment). A suitable trial would necessarily be complex and costly, and there was no pharmaceutical company to support it. Aware of the soaring expense of the ESRD program, Congress, which had created the payment program for dialysis, mandated a large trial of the low-protein diet in renal disease and funded it through the NIH and the Health Care Financing Administration (Medicare). Twelve years after the publication of Brenner's landmark paper, in the same *New England Journal of Medicine* appeared the initial report of the results of the Modification of Diet in Renal Disease Trial (MDRD).[12]

Regrettably, this complex, multimillion-dollar study produced only equivocal results. It failed to fully confirm the ability of the low-protein diet to slow progression, though it did help prove that optimal reduction of elevated blood pressure could do so. Meanwhile, also in the early 1980s a new class of drugs for hypertension appeared, known by the immense name "angiotensin-converting enzyme inhibitors," or "ACE inhibitors." The first of these, captopril, indirectly derived from substances in viper venom, won approval for general use in the United States in 1981.[13]

ACE inhibitors lessen activity of the renin-angiotensin-aldosterone pathway, a system of linked substances that play important roles in the regulation of blood pressure and the body's content of salt, water, and potassium. Excess excitement of this axis can lead to elevated blood pressure and heart failure. These drugs not only can lower blood pressure but also have been shown to relieve heart failure, improve survival after heart attacks, reduce the frequency of migraine headaches, and possibly ward off complications of diabetes and diabetes itself—truly a chosen pill for the modern man and woman, a candidate for placement in the drinking waters of urban North America and Europe, maybe India and China as well. Since angiotensin helps maintain hyperfiltration in surviving glomeruli, it was hypothesized that ACE inhibitors might

protect diseased but functioning kidneys over the long haul from
further deterioration (progression). Following favorable results in
animal studies, during the 1980s and 1990s researchers in Europe
and North America, and eventually even China, undertook large
clinical trials sponsored by government agencies and pharmaceutical companies: these confirmed that the drug could indeed slow
progression in both diabetic and nondiabetic diseases, at least for
many. Now, all the buzz in the world of renal disease centered on
progression and ACE inhibitors; with some relief, nephrologists
in the United States could give up on dietetics, about which only
a few knew very much.[14]

During the 1990s and into the 2000s, the use of ACE inhibitors to slow progression won virtually unquestioned acceptance,
though the underlying theory changed.[15] Abundant evidence suggested that ACE inhibitors worked best in slowing progression
among patients *with the most proteinuria,* which these drugs in
fact reduced. Proteinuria, not hyperfiltration, became the villain
(though the ACE inhibitors might decrease both). Worldwide,
nephrologists raised their level of attention to the protein (really
albumin) in the urine, the very phenomenon that commenced
the modern understanding of kidney disease at Guy's Hospital in
the 1820s. What had long been thought mostly a marker, or consequence, of renal disease was newly conceived as a contributor
to the injury. It is believed to happen this way: some disease such
as diabetes or FSGS (there are, of course, many others) causes a
change in the filtering surface of the glomerulus that allows passage of blood albumin across it. This albumin appears in the tubular fluid, and therefore much of the "leaked" protein will end up
in the urine. But a sizeable amount is reabsorbed—retrieved back
into the bloodstream—by the proximal tubular cells, those that
are active just beyond the glomerular outlet. According to this theory, as that albumin is taken up by these cells and passes through
them on the way back to blood capillaries, its presence within the
cells triggers an inflammatory reaction. This reaction in turn leads
to a kind of scarring (fibrosis), which eventually destroys the entire
nephron unit. As fewer nephrons remain, their abnormal glomeruli further hyperfilter, and leak even more albumin that will in
turn be taken up by their proximal tubules, with further inflam-

matory response, and so on. Thus proteinuria is now considered
not only a sign of renal disease but also a pernicious agent of its
advance.

ACE inhibitor drugs were observed to reduce proteinuria, and
by about 2000 this was considered the basis for their ability to
preserve renal function. In the 1990s, a class of medication acting
similarly to ACE inhibitors called angiotensin receptor blockers,
or ARBs, entered the formularies of the world. Soon, some investigators asserted that using the two agents together achieved even
better reduction of proteinuria and (presumably) preservation of
renal filtration than either alone. Other authorities advocated the
use of ACE inhibitors in very large doses. The nephrology journals
and lectures at national meetings began to show data charts for patients whose progression stopped altogether with the use of ACE
inhibitors and ARBs. It seemed that a few even regained some lost
kidney function.

These were encouraging, indeed at times amazing, results.
Nephrologists throughout the world by the end of the 1990s felt
confident that progression of chronic renal disease really could be
slowed, and dialysis delayed or perhaps entirely avoided, mainly
through use of these drugs. Practitioners continued to recognize
the importance as well of effective control of blood pressure, and
of blood sugar in those with diabetic renal disease. A new epide-
miologic manner of thinking drove renal specialists to talk less
about "causes" and more about "risk factors" for chronic kidney
disease or its progression. By the early twenty-first century the list
of such risk factors grew to include obesity and cigarette smoking.
But ACE inhibitors and angiotensin receptor blockers remained
the mainstays of "renoprotective" treatment. As with other treatments of Bright's Disease in the past, they carried some risk. They
could lead to potentially dangerous retention of potassium, already a worry in persons with faulty renal function. Occasionally,
a person with narrowing of the main arteries to the kidney would
experience a sudden and severe plunge in the already decreased
level of renal filtration, a picture of "acute-on-chronic" renal failure. But in general, when used judiciously, the antiangiotensin
medications proved safe and free of serious side effects. Reliance
on these drugs for the treatment of renal disease before its end

stage has further entwined the nephrology specialty and its patients with the pharmaceutical industry, though this relationship occurs with many chronic diseases. Heads of pharmaceutical companies cherish medications that large numbers of persons will take indefinitely.

And, from the point of view of nephrologists, the sooner started, the better. It seemed plausible that if these drugs can slow progression of renal disease, the maximal benefit ought to result from detecting and treating at an early stage. Every nephrology practitioner has repeatedly had the painful experience of seeing a patient for the first time who already has advanced disease, with shrunken kidneys and uremic symptoms, and in need of prompt hemodialysis. Furthermore, given the prevalence of diabetes and hypertension in Western countries, it seemed probable that there might be millions of persons "out there" with early, asymptomatic renal disease. Various estimations have projected that over ten million Americans (mostly in the older age range) have some degree of renal disease and that only a small proportion of them even know it.[16] In fact, symptoms do not occur until all but 10 or 15 percent of renal filtration capacity is gone; and (according to this viewpoint) primary physicians may fail to understand the meaning of small elevations in blood creatinine, or minor but detectable levels of albumin in a urine sample. Such persons might benefit from use of an ACE inhibitor or ARB as well as other preventive measures.

ANOTHER NEW NAME: CKD

By 2000, in the United States, leaders of the nephrology specialty and of the National Kidney Foundation had begun deliberations aimed at promoting early detection of renal disease and establishing sound guidelines for dealing with it once found. Such an approach seemed consistent with the well-established concept of treating asymptomatic disorders such as high blood pressure and hyperlipidemia in order to prevent devastating consequences. But the lay and professional leaders and advocates realized that first they had to overcome a problem with what has come to be called by both the business and nonprofit worlds "branding"—that is, as an organ, particularly as an organ capable of getting seriously sick, the kidney suffered from poor name recognition. A president of the American Society of Nephrology in his annual address at the 2002 meeting actually said: "First, we have to market kidney disease better. The people who are interested in stroke, cardiovascular disease, and cancer have done a far more effective job than we have in delivering a message to the lay population and to practicing physicians than we have accomplished."[17]

One obstacle to raising awareness about kidneys and kidney disease seemed to be the traditional language of the nephrologist, who had long referred to the general category of slowly worsening renal disorders as "chronic renal failure." Presumably few persons in the general population knew what "renal" meant, and (this is my own speculation) "failure" seemed an unattractive term that the leadership of nephrology in the United States would not want to embrace. Americans do not like failure. At the beginning of the "Executive Summary" of an important new set of guidelines for the detection and care of kidney disease, called the K/DOQI or Kidney/Dialysis Outcomes Quality Initiative, sponsored by the National Kidney Foundation, the reader sees this explanation: "Why 'kidney'?—The word 'kidney' is of Middle English origin and is immediately understood by patients, their families, providers, health care professionals, and the lay public of native English speakers. On the other hand, 'renal' and 'nephrology,' derived from Latin and Greek roots, respectively, commonly require interpretation and explanation. The Work Group [for these guidelines] and the NKF are committed to communicating in language that can be widely understood."[18]

Thus national leaders urged that the simple phrase "chronic kidney disease" shortened to CKD replace "chronic renal failure" to label long-standing and usually progressive loss of kidney filtering capacity, regardless of underlying cause. To aid the development and use of practice guidelines for treatment, CKD was stratified into five stages, the fifth or most serious indicating ESRD, the need for dialysis or transplantation. Such "staging" long had been utilized for cancer and heart disease, and "evidence-based" practice guidelines proliferated within American medicine in the 1990s, to be both applauded and deplored. The demystification and democratization of language—English in place of Greek or

Latin—coupled to practice guidelines and the new enthusiasm for prevention won acceptance almost overnight. Quite suddenly, "CKD" was everywhere on the lips of American nephrologists and their "fellows" (trainees); and only careless old-timers would occasionally refer to "chronic renal failure." Of course, since everyone in the specialty started saying "CKD" rather than the full "chronic kidney disease," other persons including patients still at first did not know what we were talking about. Some medical school nephrology groups set up CKD Clinics to administer efficient guidelines-based care. As the use of epoetin to treat the anemia of kidney disease extended to those not yet requiring dialysis, nephrologists found themselves carrying out injections of this drug, and infusing new iron preparations into patients, while learning to talk and teach about the nuances of blood formation.[19] We became the objects of an enormous onslaught of attention and advertising from the manufacturers of the iron solutions, as they joined the makers of epoetin, ACE inhibitors and ARBs, and phosphate binders.[20]

As noted above, certain estimates projected that ten million or more Americans alone might have some degree of CKD and might benefit from early preventive measures. Renal specialists proposed that many such persons could be identified at an early stage, mainly by checking blood creatinine as part of periodic health screening and plugging the value into an equation that yields a kidney filtration rate.[21] Early detection and treatment became the central motivation for the Chronic Kidney Disease Initiative launched in 2004 under the auspices of the Council of American Kidney Societies.[22] The overall objective was to improve CKD outcomes; "outcomes," like "guidelines," was another word that seemed everywhere in the rhetoric of American medicine of the late 1990s and early twenty-first century. For CKD, improving outcomes meant avoiding or delaying ESRD, as well as avoiding or minimizing complications of chronic kidney disease, such as the anemia and deterioration of bones discussed in earlier chapters.

By 2000, considerable evidence also indicated that chronic renal disease counted as a substantial risk factor for heart disease. Those attending the planning workshop for the CKD Initiative included nephrologists and nurses from private practice and medical schools, one patient, and representatives from: the NIH, a large health maintenance organization, Medicare, the dialysis industry, a national laboratory company, foundations, health policy institutes, and four pharmaceutical companies. These "Stakeholder Sectors" amply demonstrated how Bright's Disease, under whatever new name, had come to dwell in an interlocking array of components making up the medical-industrial-governmental complex of modern technological medicine. I have pointed this out before in the context of ESRD and dialysis, and the relationship would apply as well to other major chronic diseases, but none more so than those of the kidneys.

Some readers will not comfortably see the CKD Initiative as anything but self-serving. Is it not merely a manifestation of the "identity politics" of big diseases, a strategy for increasing research funding, referrals, and (for pharmaceutical companies) the sale of medicines? And what about translating slightly high readings of a single blood test (creatinine) from the autoanalyzers of America, by way of a computerized equation, into millions of cases of pre-symptomatic kidney disease?[23] Isn't this merely more medicalization of the well, disease boosterism, driven by too much authority ceded to the medical establishment, and too much profit-seeking within the drug industry? It would be naïve to discount such perceptions. I can say, as a still-practicing nephrologist as I write this (if now only a small part of my time), that most of us do abhor the idea that all persons with some degree of renal injury must necessarily get worse and end up needing dialysis or transplantation. The application of risk-factor reduction and the use of drugs acting on the renin-angiotensin-aldosterone pathway do seem effective in preserving kidney function, at least for many, and, as already noted, nothing has attracted as much attention at nephrology conventions and in our publications for the last decade.

Whatever one might think of the CKD Initiative and the notion that ten million or more unsuspecting Americans have underperforming kidneys, the movement has spread vigorously. A president of the International Society of Nephrology (ISN) referred to the "new nephrology": "All core ISN programs . . . have been expanded and restructured to emphasize early detection and prevention."[24] The International Federation of Kidney Foundations and the ISN have declared the need for a World Kidney Day. It is to be "fully inaugurated" on Thursday, March 8, 2007 (and presumably was, as these words are read). "The aim is to broadcast the message about kidney disease to government health officials, general physicians, allied health professionals, individuals, and families." The committee for World Kidney Day wants to see more attention to "detection and prevention" not just in North America and Europe but throughout the world. The goal is to achieve "a major reduction in the global burden of kidney and cardiovascular disease."[25] The theme of World Kidney Day for 2007 was to be "Get to Know Your Kidneys." I admitted in introducing this book that no one writes songs about the kidneys, but with a World Kidney Day, maybe the time will come.

I've chosen to pay attention to the names given to diffuse kidney disease and how they reflect their medical culture. "Dropsy" (which was not always renal in origin) was disease as symptom, apparent to patient, family, and doctor. "Bright's Disease" in the 1820s to 1830s announced a new way of defining disease, based on findings invisible to the ill person—alterations in internal organs, revealed at autopsy, chemical changes in blood or urine. Terms such as "glomerulonephritis" or "focal segmental glomerulosclerosis" appeared when those trying to classify and understand disease turned to the microscope, and eventually the biopsy needle, to tease out subtle distinctions. "ESRD" came along, in the United States, as a bureaucratic label for totally failed kidneys, entitling their owner to reimbursement for replacement therapy with another new technology, the artificial kidney, or transplantation. "CKD," or "chronic kidney disease," was consciously selected as a clear and general phrase to encompass all levels of impaired kidney function regardless of the more specific underlying disorder that caused the injury. Like Bright's Disease, a diagnosis of CKD can be applied merely on the basis of an abnormal laboratory finding—albumin in the urine (the finding Bright explored) or an elevated blood creatinine content (which Thomas Addis advocated as a tool later in his career). CKD is diagnosed in the individual, but it is the first of these names that purposely looks toward large populations, with an epidemiological foundation—the "burden" of millions of CKD cases, the need for a public health "initiative" to address it.

—◦◦◦◦—

During the second half of the twentieth century, it has become an accepted belief that the story of human disease can best be told in the context not just of scientific thought and clinical practice but also its social and cultural setting. Similarly, disease, seemingly an inevitable part of human life, can serve as a revealing probe in understanding the workings of society. These approaches are exemplified in the works of historians such as Erwin Ackerknecht, Owsei Temkin, Charles Rosenberg, Roy Porter, and their numerous students and followers. So it is with Bright's Disease, or generalized kidney disease, regardless of the current term. Both the physician and the patient, and indeed the disease, have resided in physical and social places, places that have changed and grown. So, all three have made journeys.

From the *physician's* perspective, the job has been creating knowledge about underlying structural change (pathology), cause, and mechanism, and devising treatments. Physicians moved from the bedside, to the autopsy room, then microscope bench and laboratory to build the categorization and understanding. For example, the syndrome of acute renal failure newly recognized in the 1930s stimulated a huge amount of work in the animal laboratory, using rats and other animals to create experimental models of the disorder. Clinician-researchers included in this volume, like Thomas Addis and Barry Brenner, but many others as well throughout the world, assembled laboratory teams in order to understand the progressive, downhill behavior of chronic kidney disease. Others have studied the mechanisms associated with proteinuria. Quite separately from the fastidious laboratory groups, it was mostly surgeons working alone who sought to simply go ahead and replace the function of failed kidneys with a machine or a transplant. Their destination was a room that could serve as tinkerer's shop, sometimes in a basement, or the dog laboratory, in which to try out transplant techniques. Remarkably, both efforts—to build a kidney and to transplant a kidney—won eventual success well before similar measures aided people with non-working hearts or livers. In a period that increasingly honored medicine and adored technology, affluent societies managed to establish complex systems to provide these emblematic products of the twentieth century. Prevention, and the ancient remedy of adjusting diet, were for many years easily displaced by dialysis and transplantation until the rise of a "new nephrology."

I hope I have shown from the *patient's* perspective how kidney disease and its treatments over time could alter the lived life, as any serious illness can do. I did not know until I was well into writing this book that I would find myself struck with how dropsy and kidney disease had the capacity to stimulate travel, or at least the idea of it. We have seen Henry Fielding going to Portugal; Richard Bright's and William Osler's recommendations of removal to a warm climate; the dialysis patient on the van three times a week or sometimes driving fifty miles to the center; and kidneys and recipients rendezvousing at a metropolitan transplant center. It is true that in life and in art taking to bed signifies the shift from wellness to illness, and of course this too can occur with kidney disease. But sometimes it can be taking to the road, with its risks and opportunities. We might imagine a transhistorical renal patient making other journeys as well—from receiving drugs and tappings of the dropsical belly at home; to the hospital (and sometimes its morgue) as a newly identified victim of "albuminuric dropsy" or Bright's Disease, perhaps a potential contributor of a "granular kidney" to the museum collection. Most recently, we imagine our renal everypatient early in her illness attending a CKD Clinic in the company of many others who give blood and take pills for a disease that is not yet an illness.

Until working on this book, I had not anticipated the persisting importance of returning to work as the marker of success or failure in the treatment of renal disease—though this has been obvious to students of other chronic diseases. Obviously, the ability to work equals economic capability and, for most persons, confers a normal role within society. The emphasis placed on getting back to work by the physicians encountered in this volume, all of them men, no doubt reveals gendered assumptions, the equating of identity and worth with visible work outside the house. But women who were mainly homemakers could also feel the devastation of being disabled by a chronic ailment or its imperfect therapy. Disease can, of course, profoundly alter a person's outlook and viewpoints in ways unrelated to work. It can generate fear, anger, and despair. As we saw with dialysis and transplantation, however, it can also provide the setting or opportunity for moral choices, valor, selflessness, and even an affirmation of Divine reality in one's life. This amounts to another form of movement, an unexpected transition brought on by sickness in the kidneys.

The experience of having kidney disease or receiving one of its treatments, at least in the United States, has come to be embedded in a complex set of arrangements and structures, physical and organizational. These include medicine and hospitals but also governments, suppliers of equipment, pharmaceutical companies, foundations, health insurers, and advocacy organizations. We have produced variants of this list several times; here we might add for good measure the electricity grid, the media, and surely the Internet, where people with renal disease find information and share their stories. Even amateur and professional sports for some patients factor into the experience of losing kidney function. Participants in what I will call the enterprise of kidney disease and its treatments, beyond patients, nurses, and doctors, include laboratory and dialysis technicians, social workers, pharmacists, tissue typers, van drivers, legislators, factory workers making filters and medications, clerks, newsletter editors, publicists, and the list goes on. Such lists merely reflect, one might say, our existence in the *non*-diseased life of the twenty-first century—the various "grids" and systems we rely upon each day. (And that is part of the point—life with disease is enabled and shaped by the arrangements of a particular society.) But the person who goes for hemodialysis treatments three times in a week is more critically dependent than most persons on the unseen workings of the electric company and on the availability of some open, moving lanes on the freeway. Indeed, one can assert that it is not merely the dialysis filter or transplanted organ that replaces the work of failed kidneys, but in fact the whole apparatus of systems and personnel.

Yet, the history of dropsy and kidney disease reveals as well the persisting meaning and importance of particular human connections. In one sense, anyone who is sick suffers alone, since no one else can feel that person's singular discomfort and fear. But in probably all cultures, illness is more or less an intimately shared experience, involving in some ways family, friends, healers, and others. We might recall Henry Fielding's requirement for a captain who would finally get his ship moving toward Portugal, and for a surgeon willing to visit on board to carry out paracentesis, and— most poignantly—for his wife and family, who accompanied him on the futile voyage in search of a cure. The diagnosis of Bright's Disease in Lydia Cassatt raised fear in her close-knit family and altered its dynamics. As her malady made her less a participant in family events, she became the tranquil subject for the growing portraiture skills of her sister Mary. An enduring friendship, supported by shared intellect and political viewpoints, arose from the clinical relationship of doctor Tom Addis, his patient Linus Pauling, and Pauling's wife Ava Helen, who became deputy physician. Hemodialysis at a large center may seem impersonal, yet friendships develop among patients during the slow hours on the machine, as well as bonding between patients and their nurses, physicians, and technicians. It is usually a spouse or family member who assists the person doing dialysis at home. The experience of kidney donation has created literally unprecedented forms of human relationships between relatives or between friends, and in so doing has extended the concepts of gift, altruism, and possibly obligation.

Both the patient's experience of kidney disease and medical ways of understanding it point out something easily overlooked in historical narratives—namely, continuities over time. Paracentesis for relieving dropsy spans at least two millennia in Western medicine; it is still done in 2006. People also still take diuretic pills, and they or their physician pinch the ankles in search of pitting.[26] Proteinuria persists in importance both as diagnostic signifier of renal disease but now also as a probable factor in its evolution within a patient's body. Although I have called attention to the modern grids and systems in which renal disease and its treatments now exist, one might argue that even in Richard Bright's time the care of his patients at Guy's Hospital, which contained over four hundred beds in the 1820s, depended upon a sizeable staff and bureaucracy to make such an institution work. Merely getting supplies into and waste out of such an institution each day offered challenges. Beyond this, Bright's ability to delineate albuminuric kidney disease and make that work known required the contributions of pupils, chemical- and pathology-minded colleagues, painters, engravers, colorists, typesetters, editors, and publishers. Perhaps one of the most striking continuities in the story of kidney disease is the recent return to reliance on a broad name and concept—Bright's Disease has in effect been reborn as CKD.

Bright, as an "advocate" for the importance of the disease he had defined, asserted in an 1836 article that it was "among the most frequent, as well as most certain causes of death in some classes of the community " and a "common occurrence in all." He estimated that "not less than five hundred die of it annually in London alone."[27] Leaders of the defined specialty called nephrology in the early twenty-first century have similarly voiced alarms about the prevalence and consequences of kidney disease. They have prescribed plans for early detection of such disease and have codified treatments to avoid or slow its progression and to lessen its damaging effects elsewhere in the body. In furtherance of these new objectives, medical and advocacy organizations created the CKD Initiative and proclaim a "new nephrology." But in the nephrology journals and at our meetings, we hear very little about how these efforts to find and treat millions might be supported financially. In the United States, ESRD care (dialysis and transplantation) was costing government, insurance plans, and patients well over $20 billion annually by the year 2000. Identifying the purported ten million or more Americans with early CKD and treating most with the appropriate drugs to slow progression, and some with epoetin and iron, would of course prove enormously expensive. Even the massive expenditure on ESRD care alone raises questions about allocation of resources—though there would seem to be no going back.

Furthermore, there remain imperfections and unanswered questions surrounding both dialysis and transplantation, so research in these areas cannot be abandoned. Nor should research into the fundamental causes and mechanisms of renal disease: recall that the recent progress has been in *secondary* prevention, the attempt to avoid worsening of disease already present, not in true "primary" prevention of the disease. On a global basis, serious kidney disease occurs in large part from malaria, schistosomiasis, AIDS, and other infectious diseases in parts of the world little able to deal adequately with the primary disorder, much less the renal complications. And, even a World Kidney Day will hardly defeat the competing claims of heart disease or cancer for attention and funding.

When Bright's Disease or ESRD afflicts and changes individuals, it does so within the strata of social settings. Kidney disease considered epidemiologically (e.g., as CKD) functions as well within economic and political environments. Nephrologists speak of the healthy kidney as the organ of the body that ensures certain essential forms of chemical "balance," meaning something like correct quantities and proportions.[28] We refer to "acid-base balance" or "salt and water balance"—it is the latter that has gone wrong in the person with dropsy. The dominant questions for the future of kidney disease will be ones of balance. Can governmental budgets balance the desire to effect prevention in the early phase of disease with the need to provide replacement treatment for its terminal stage? How might the value of detecting CKD in its earliest phase be weighed against the emotional and economic costs of declaring tens of millions of people diseased based on a single blood test and equation? What would be needed to see industry still contribute beneficial drugs and devices without overly influencing medical practice and medical education, or amassing unseemly profits? How well can physicians and nurses remain attuned to the emotional as well as medical needs of individuals with renal disease while functioning within an increasingly "epidemiological" framework that stresses large numbers? These are not, of course, questions unique to the kidney in our era of chronic disease. But Bright's Disease—ESRD, CKD—has over many years earned the full right to ask them.

NOTES

Preface

1. Steven J. Peitzman, "Nephrology in America from Thomas Addis to the Artificial Kidney," in Russell C. Maulitz and Diana E. Long, eds., *Grand Rounds: One Hundred Years of Internal Medicine in America* (Philadelphia: University of Pennsylvania Press, 1988), 211–41 (an earlier version appeared as "Nephrology in the United States from Osler to the Artificial Kidney," *Annals of Internal Medicine* 105 [1986]: 937–46); idem, "Science, Inventors, and the Introduction of the Artificial Kidney in the United States," *Seminars in Dialysis* 9 (1996): 276–81; idem, "Chronic Dialysis and Dialysis Doctors in the United States: A Nephrologist-Historian's Perspective," *Seminars in Dialysis* 14 (2001): 200–208.

2. A useful source for the "premolecular" era is Carl W. Gottschalk, Robert W. Berliner, and Gerhard H. Giebisch, eds., *Renal Physiology: People and Ideas* (Bethesda, Md.: American Physiological Society, 1987).

Chapter 1. Swollen with Dropsy

1. John Wesley, *Primitive Physic, or an Easy and Natural Method of Curing Most Diseases,* introduction by A. Wesley Hill (London: Epworth Press, 1960; reprint of the 23rd edition, 1791), 63; H. P. Cholmeley, *John of Gaddesden and the Rosa Medicinae* (Oxford: Clarendon Press, 1912), 29.

2. Frederik Dekkers, *Exercitationes Practicae circa Medendi Methodum, Auctoritate, Ratione, Observationibusve Plurimis Confirmatae ac Figuris Illustratae* (Leyden, 1695). The woodcut is opposite p. 290, the case narrative on pp. 285–91.

3. Thomas Sydenham, *A Treatise of the Gout and Dropsy,* in *The Works of Thomas Sydenham on Acute and Chronic Diseases,* annotated by George Wallis (London, 1788), vol. 2, 260.

4. William Withering, *An Account of the Foxglove and Some of Its Medical Uses: With Practical Remarks on Dropsy, and other Diseases* (Birmingham, 1785), 87.

5. E. D. Phillips, *Aspects of Greek Medicine* (Philadelphia: The Charles Press, 1987; first published as *Greek Medicine* in 1973), 154.

6. Cholmeley, *John of Gaddesden,* 36–37.

7. Robert V. Remini, *Andrew Jackson and the Course of American Democracy, 1833–1845* (New York: Harper and Row, 1984), vol. 3, 519.

8. Philostratus, *The Life of Appolonius of Tyana,* ed. and trans. Christopher P. Jones (Cambridge, Mass.: Harvard University Press, 2005), 49; Sydenham, *Treatise of the Gout and Dropsy,* 264; William Cullen, *First Lines of the Practice of Physic* (Edinburgh, 1787), vol. 4, 259; William Buchan, *Domestic Medicine or, A Treatise*

on the Prevention and Cure of Diseases by Regimen and Simple Medicines, 9th ed. (Dublin, 1784), 299; John Dunn Hunter, *Memoirs of a Captivity Among the Indians of North America,* 3rd ed. (London: Longman's, 1824), 438. See also: Daniel Drake, *A Discourse on Intemperance* (Cincinnati: Looker and Reynold Printers, 1828), 40–41 (intemperance can cause dropsy); George Gregory, *A Lecture on Dropsy* (London: Burgess and Hill, 1819), 24–26 (dropsy following heavy drinking "is another every day occurrence").

9. Samuel Johnson, *The Letters of Samuel Johnson,* ed. R. W. Chapman (Oxford: Clarendon Press, 1952), vol. 3, 131.

10. Ibid., 133.

11. Ibid., 136.

12. Ibid., 186.

13. Ibid., 185.

14. Ibid., 217.

15. Ibid., 236.

16. Ibid., 247.

17. Ibid., 198.

18. Ibid., 247–48.

19. William Heberden, *Commentaries on the History and Cure of Diseases* (1802; facsimile reprint edition, New York: Library of the New York Academy of Medicine and Hafner Publishing Co., 1962), 216.

20. See, e.g., Thomas Forbes, "By What Disease or Casualty: The Changing Face of Death in London," in Charles Webster, ed., *Health, Medicine and Mortality in the Sixteenth Century* (Cambridge: Cambridge University Press, 1979), 117–39.

21. J. Worth Estes, *Hall Jackson and the Purple Foxglove* (Hanover, N.H.: University Press of New England, 1979), esp. 143–46 (dropsy mortality).

22. For discussion about the causation of dropsy, see Phillips, *Aspects of Greek Medicine;* Alain Touwaide and Natale Gaspare De Santo, "Edema in the Corpus Hippocraticum," *American Journal of Nephrology* 19 (1999): 155–58; Donald Monro, *An Essay on the Dropsy and Its Different Species,* 2nd ed. (London, 1756); Sydenham, *Treatise of the Gout and Dropsy;* Cullen, *First Lines;* Saul Jarcho, *The Concept of Heart Failure* (Cambridge, Mass.: Harvard University Press, 1980); J. Worth Estes, "Dropsy," in Kenneth Kiple, ed., *The Cambridge World History of Human Disease* (Cambridge: Cambridge University Press, 1993), 689–96. Dropsy was also considered a cold, phlegmatic disease by French practitioners; see Lawrence Brockliss and Colin Jones, *The Medical World of Early Modern France* (Oxford: Clarendon Press, 1997), 114, 154.

23. See, e.g., Cholmeley, *John of Gaddesden* (discussion of dropsy), and Richard Wiseman, *Eight Surgical Treatises,* 3rd ed. (London, 1697), 123.

24. For dropsy remedies in American almanacs, see Thomas Horrocks, "Rules, Remedies and Regimens: Almanacs and Popular Medicine in Early America" (PhD diss., University of Pennsylvania, 2003), 81–91.

25. This case and the phrases quoted are found in Sydenham, *Treatise of the Gout and Dropsy,* 284–85.

26. For this idea of a jointly agreed-upon therapeutic action, see Charles Rosen-

berg, "The Therapeutic Revolution," in *Explaining Epidemics and Other Studies in the History of Medicine* (Cambridge: Cambridge University Press, 1992), 9–31.

27. Historians tend to frown upon these sorts of retrospective judgments of the possible validity of historical therapeutic measures, rightly preferring to understand practice within the context of its own time. The "Later Perspective" sections at the end of chapters 1–6 are aimed to separate outdated from still-relevant ideas and practices and to provide some brief understandings of thought in nephrology at the time of this writing.

28. Withering, *Account of the Foxglove,* 2.

29. Ibid., 9.

30. Ibid., 25–26.

31. Ibid., 58.

32. Henry Fielding, *The Journal of a Voyage to Lisbon,* ed. with intro. and notes by Tom Keymer (London: Penguin Books, 1996; first published 1755), 17.

33. Ibid., 18.

34. Ibid., 19–20.

35. Ibid., 20.

36. Ibid., 30. Presumably Fielding refers to William Hunter (1718–1783), anatomist, surgeon, and later in his career, prominent obstetrician.

37. Ibid., 93.

38. Remini, *Andrew Jackson,* 521.

39. Wiseman, *Eight Surgical Treatises,* 123.

40. *Gentleman's Magazine* 2 (January 1732): 585.

41. *Gentleman's Magazine* 7 (September 1737): 573. These may have been cases of ovarian cysts.

42. George M. Gould and Walter L. Pyle, *Anomalies and Curiosities of Medicine* (Philadelphia: Saunders, 1897), 786.

43. F. Salerno, M. Merli, O. Riggio, M. Cazzaniga, V. Valeriano, M. Pozzi, A. Nicolini, F. Salvatori, "Randomized Controlled Study of TIPS Versus Paracentesis Plus Albumin in Cirrhosis with Severe Ascites," *Hepatology* 40 (2004): 629–35.

Chapter 2. Richard Bright's New Disease

1. Ralph Josselin, *The Diary of Ralph Josselin* (London: The British Academy, 1976), 643 ("I was very ill, and concluded by the swelling of my thighs and belly it was the dropsy"); *Gentleman's Magazine* 21 (1751): 326; e.g., "The trembling knees no more sustain / The water's weight above / And smit [*sic*] together tried in vain / The load below to move"; George Eliot, *The Mill on the Floss,* ed. Gordon Haight (Oxford: Oxford University Press, 1996), 57–58.

2. The full title is *Reports of Medical Cases, Selected with a View of Illustrating the Symptoms and Cure of Diseases by A Reference to Morbid Anatomy* (London: Longman, Rees, Orme, Brown & Green, 1827–1831). It was published as two volumes in three quartos. The sections dealing with kidney disease have been reprinted in *Original Papers of Richard Bright on Renal Disease,* ed. A. Arnold Osman (London: Oxford University Press, 1937), 1–92; and in William B. Ober, ed., *Great Men of Guy's* (Metuchen, N.J.: Scarecrow Reprint Corp., 1973), 63–162.

3. Pamela Bright, *Dr. Richard Bright (1789–1858)* (London: Bodley Head, 1983), 140.

4. Edmond Arnold, "Medical Reminiscences," *Atlanta Medical Weekly* 8 (1897): 325–31, quote on p. 331.

5. The expert on color printing was Joan Friedman, who in the 1970s, when she graciously helped the author, was Rare Books Curator at the Yale Center for British Art. Christine Ruggere, now with the Institute for the History of Medicine at Johns Hopkins University, helped me understand the business ledgers for the *Reports of Medical Cases* when I began to study the history of the book. For more on the production of the *Reports of Medical Cases,* see Steven J. Peitzman, "Bright's Disease and Bright's Generation—Toward Exact Medicine at Guy's Hospital," *Bulletin of the History of Medicine* 55 (1981): 307–21.

6. One perceives the same purpose, and many of the same techniques, in the great illustrated books of birds and plants produced in Britain and elsewhere in the first half of the nineteenth century. Audubon's *Birds of North America* was produced in England, using methods very similar to those Bright selected for the *Reports of Medical Cases.*

7. The full Latin title of Harvey's book is *Anatomica Exercitatio de Motu Cordis & Sanguinis in Animalibus* (in English, *Anatomical Exercises [or Disquisition] on the Motion of the Heart and Blood in Animals;* Giovanni Battista Morgagni, *De Sedibus, et Causis Morborum per Anatomen Indagatis; Libri Quinque* (Venetiis: Ex typographia Remondiniana, 1761); Matthew Baillie, *The Morbid Anatomy of Some of the Most Important Parts of the Human Body* (London: J. Johnson, 1793).

8. Some of the essential works on anatomy, pathology, and medicine in France during this period are: Erwin Ackerknecht, *Medicine in the Paris Hospital, 1794–1848* (Baltimore: Johns Hopkins University Press, 1966); Owsei Temkin, "The Role of Surgery in the Rise of Modern Medical Thought," *Bulletin of the History of Medicine* 25 (1951): 248–59; Russell Maulitz, *Morbid Appearances* (Cambridge: Cambridge University Press, 1987); John Harley Warner, *Against the Spirit of System: The French Impulse in Nineteenth-Century American Medicine* (Princeton: Princeton University Press, 1998). There exists as well an enormous and still-growing journal literature on French medicine in this period.

9. There exist two biographies of Richard Bright. Pamela Bright's *Dr. Richard Bright (1789–1858),* already cited, utilizes many family letters and is strong on Bright the individual and his relationships with his family. *Richard Bright 1789–1858: Physician in an Age of Revolution and Reform,* by Diana Berry and Campbell Mackenzie (London: Royal Society of Medicine Services, Ltd., 1992) is stronger concerning Bright's medical and pathological work.

10. Bright, *Reports of Medical Cases,* 2.

11. Ibid., 7.

12. Ibid., 29–30.

13. Ibid., 31.

14. Ibid., 71.

15. Richard Bright, "Cases and Observations Illustrative of Renal Disease Ac-

companied with the Secretion of Albuminous Urine," *Guy's Hospital Reports* 1 (1836): 338–79, "history of this disease" on pp. 338–41.

16. See Steven J. Peitzman, "From Bright's Disease to End-Stage Renal Disease," in *Framing Disease: Studies in Cultural History* (New Brunswick, N.J.: Rutgers University Press, 1992), 3–32.

17. Thomas Watson, *Lectures on the Principles and Practice of Physic* (Philadelphia: Lea and Blanchard, 1844), 779.

18. Bright, "Cases and Observations," 356.

19. Lydia Cassatt was diagnosed with Bright's Disease, though the family at times did not accept that opinion. She did die in her forties from some chronic, remitting disease, marked by fatigue, nausea and vomiting, and pain. The letter is quoted in Nancy Hale, *Mary Cassatt* (New York: Doubleday, 1975), 77. A novel appeared in 2001 that imaginatively explores the relationship between sisters Lydia and Mary, and the centrality of Lydia's Bright's Disease in shaping that relationship: Harriet Scott Chessman, *Lydia Cassatt Reading the Morning Paper* (New York: The Permanent Press and Seven Stories Press, 2001).

20. John R. Bumgarner, *The Health of the Presidents* (Jefferson, N.C.: McFarland & Co., 1994), 133.

21. Daniel W. Cathell, *The Physician Himself and What He Should Add to the Strictly Scientific* (Baltimore: Cushings & Bailey, 1882), 82. This compilation of sensible advice and cynicism went through many editions.

22. Nancy Mowll Mathews, *Mary Cassatt: A Life* (New York: Villard Books, 1994), 160–61.

23. Historian Charles Rosenberg in his recent publications and lectures has been considering the various "powers" and meanings of the disease entity, especially as applied to a person within a society. See, e.g., his "The Tyranny of Diagnosis: Specific Entities and Individual Experience," *Milbank Quarterly* 80 (2002): 237–60. Susan Sontag began her esteemed essay "Illness as Metaphor" by stating: "Illness is the night-side of life, a more onerous citizenship. Everyone who is born holds dual citizenship, in the kingdom of the well and in the kingdom of the sick." Sontag, *Illness as Metaphor and AIDS and Its Metaphors* (New York: Doubleday Anchor Books, 1990), 3. *Illness as Metaphor* was first published in 1978.

24. For the formation and early years of the Guy's Hospital School of Medicine, and reform at Guy's, see H. C. Cameron, *Mr. Guy's Hospital, 1726–1948* (London: Longmans, Green and Co., 1954), esp. 105–87.

25. For early clinical chemistry in Britain, see Noel Coley, "Medical Chemistry at Guy's Hospital (1770–1850)," *Ambix* 35 (1988): 155–68; idem, "Medical Chemists and the Origins of Clinical Chemistry in Britain (circa 1750–1850)," *Clinical Chemistry* 50 (2004): 961–72. For the shift from a pictorial to chemical and quantitative approach to the study of renal disease at Guy's, see Steven J. Peitzman, "Bright's Disease and Bright's Generation—Toward Exact Medicine at Guy's Hospital," *Bulletin of the History of Medicine* 55 (1981): 307–21.

26. Bright, *Reports of Medical Cases,* 83.

27. George H. Barlow, "Account of Observations Made Under the Superinten-

dence of Dr. Bright on Patients Whose Urine Was Albuminous, with a Chemical Examination of the Blood and Secretions by G. O. Rees, M.D.," *Guy's Hospital Reports* Ser. 2, 1 (1843): 189–330, quotation from Bright's introduction, p. 189.

28. Ibid., 189–90.

29. Ibid., 293.

30. This has been seen with AIDS, and most clearly with new diseases whose attributes suggest an infectious basis, such as Legionnaire's disease in 1976, and severe acute respiratory syndrome, or SARS, in 2002. Then, the new disease can be processed using familiar ideas and established techniques.

Chapter 3. Sympathy and Flannel

1. Richard Bright, "On the Functions of the Abdomen, and Some of the Diagnostic Marks of Its Disease" (Gulstonian Lectures, 1833. Lecture II), *London Medical Gazette* 12 (1833): 378–84, quote on pp. 380–81.

2. Richard Bright, "Cases and Observations Illustrative of Renal Disease Accompanied with Secretion of Albuminous Urine," *Guy's Hospital Reports* 1 (1836): 338–79, quote from p. 371.

3. For Bright's understanding and treatment of the disease, see Steven J. Peitzman, "Richard Bright and Mercury as the Cause and Cure of Nephritis," *Bulletin of the History of Medicine* 52 (1978): 419–43.

4. Richard Bright, *Reports of Medical Cases, Selected with a View of Illustrating the Symptoms and Cure of Diseases by A Reference to Morbid Anatomy* (London: Longman, Rees, Orme, Brown & Green, 1827–1831). The cases cited are from vol. 1. For reprinted excerpts that might be more readily available, see note 2 for chapter 2.

5. Bright, "Cases and Observations," 356.

6. John Chadwick and W. N. Mann, *The Medical Works of Hippocrates* (Oxford: Blackwell, 1950), 60, 79.

7. There exists, of course, an enormous historical literature on the moral meaning of illness and epidemics, even if one sets aside sexually transmitted diseases and disorders of the mind. Some examples, representing several generations of medical historians writing in English, and a variety of approaches, would include: Owsei Temkin, "Medicine and the Problem of Moral Responsibility," in his *The Double Face of Janus and Other Essays in the History of Medicine* (Baltimore: Johns Hopkins University Press, 1977), 50–67; Charles Rosenberg, *The Cholera Years* (Chicago: University of Chicago Press, 1987; first published 1962); Roy Porter and G. S. Rousseau, *Gout: The Patrician Malady* (New Haven, Conn.: Yale University Press, 1998); Keith Wailoo, "'Chlorosis' Remembered," in his *Drawing Blood: Technology and Disease Identity in Twentieth-Century America* (Baltimore: Johns Hopkins University Press, 1997), 17–45.

8. A pleuritic chest pain is sharp and is felt with each breath, and with coughing. Indicators of inflammation that Bright and his co-workers saw when examining the internal membranous "lining" surfaces of the body included redness, bleeding and oozing, thickening, and the appearance of certain deposits.

9. Bright, *Reports of Medical Cases*, 29–31.

10. In cupping, a small glass cup is heated in a certain manner to extrude air

and create a partial vacuum. The cup is then placed mouth-down over an area of skin that has been scarified, or cut. The vacuum will draw out a limited amount of blood. It was believed that cupping locally (say, over the heart) could relieve symptoms originating at that location. William Harvey's demonstration of the circulation of the blood in the early seventeenth century did not, somehow, shake the belief in local cupping over the next two hundred years.

11. Bright, *Reports of Medical Cases,* 31.

12. Bright, "Cases and Observations," 378–79.

13. Ibid., 372–73.

14. See René Dubos and Jean Dubos, *The White Plague* (New Brunswick, N.J.: Rutgers University Press, 1987; first published in 1952), 11–27; Sheila M. Rothman, *Living in the Shadow of Death: Tuberculosis and the Social Experience of Illness in American History* (Baltimore: Johns Hopkins University Press, 1994), 26–44; for therapeutic travels in the United States, mainly in relation to lung disease, see Carla Christine Keirns, "Short of Breath: A Social and Intellectual History of Asthma in the United States" (PhD diss., University of Pennsylvania, 2004), 81–117.

15. Richard Bright, "Cases and Observations Illustrative of Renal Disease Accompanied with the Secretion of Albuminous Urine. Memoir the Second." *Guy's Hospital Reports* 5 (1840): 101–61. The case here described is found on pp. 110–13.

16. The 1892 cases are from John M. Swan, "Case Reports on a Great Variety of Ailments Observed at Philadelphia General Hospital and University Hospital, 1890–1893," bound manuscript in·two volumes, Library of the College of Physicians of Philadelphia. Tyson authored *A Treatise on Bright's Disease and Diabetes, with Especial Reference to Pathology and Therapeutics* (Philadelphia: Lindsay and Blakiston, 1881); the lady who felt well in Germany is described on p. 186.

17. William Osler, *The Principles and Practice of Medicine,* 6th ed. (New York: Appleton, 1905), 700–702.

Chapter 4. Enter the Microscope and the Laboratory

1. Rayer was one of the earliest and most important students of Bright's Disease after Bright. He compiled an enormous treatise on diseases of the kidney and urinary tract, *Traité des Maladies des Reins et des Altérations de la Sécrétion Urinaire, Etudiées en Elles-memes et dans leurs Rapports avec les Maladies des Uretères, de la Vessie, de la Prostate de l'Urèthre,* etc. (Paris: Baillière, 1837–1841). It included a monumental colored atlas.

2. *Reports of Medical Cases, Selected with a View of Illustrating the Symptoms and Cure of Diseases by A Reference to Morbid Anatomy* (London: Longman, Rees, Orme, Brown & Green, 1827–1831), 67–70. The large, red kidney would have been that seen in what later became known as acute glomerulonephritis. Bright also shows, in his plate 4, a seemingly large, pale kidney not fitting into his three categories, which in retrospect would be considered the "large white kidney" of what became known as nephrotic syndrome, defined later in chapter 4.

3. Erwin Ackerknecht, *A Short History of Medicine* (Baltimore: Johns Hopkins University Press, 1982), 157–61; W. D. Foster, *A Short History of Clinical Pathology* (Edinburgh: Livingstone, 1961), 11–33. The "cell theory" is the broad term assigned to

the idea that all living entities consist of cells and that, in medicine, altered structure and function can be reduced to the level of the cell.

4. For details, see Carl Bartels, "Diseases of the Kidney," in H. von Ziemssen, *Cyclopedia of the Practice of Medicine,* trans. Reginald Southey and Robert Bertolet, Albert H. Buck ed. of American edition (New York: William Wood, 1877), vol. 15, 163–89; James Tyson, *Treatise on Bright's Disease and Diabetes* (Philadelphia: Lindsay and Blakiston, 1881), 79–84.

5. Friedrich Theodor von Frerichs, *Die Bright'sche Nierenkrankheit und deren Behandlung* (Braunschweig: F. Vieweg und sohn, 1851).

6. Rudolph Virchow, *Cellular Pathology,* trans. from 2nd ed. by Frank Chance (London: John Churchill, 1860), 379–82. "Parenchymatous" refers to the active, cellular content of the kidney, "interstitial" to a sort of background material in which the cellular structures exist. "Amyloid" is discussed later in chapter 4.

7. George Johnson, *Lectures on Bright's Disease* (London: Smith Elder, 1873).

8. Franz Volhard and Theodor Fahr, *Die Brightsche Nierenkrankheit* (Berlin: Springer, 1914).

9. Thomas Addis, *The Renal Lesion in Bright's Disease* (New York: Hoeber, 1931).

10. For a clear statement of a representative classification in the mid–1920s, see Herman Elwyn, *Nephritis* (New York: MacMillan, 1926), esp. 67–78.

11. Knud Faber, *Nosography: The Evolution of Clinical Medicine in Modern Times,* 2nd ed. (New York: Hoeber, 1930), 211.

12. Gout is now considered a form of acute and very painful arthritis caused by excess uric acid that sets up an inflammation in joints, particularly those of the big toe and knee.

13. Tyson, *Treatise on Bright's Disease,* 166.

14. William Osler, *The Principles and Practice of Medicine,* 6th ed. (New York: Appleton, 1905), 695.

15. Golding Bird, *Urinary Deposits: Their Diagnosis, Pathology, and Therapeutical Indications* (London: Churchill, 1844); James Tyson, *Guide to the Practical Examination of Urine for the Use of Physicians and Students* (Philadelphia: Lindsay and Blakiston, 1875).

16. As would renal biopsy beginning in the late 1940s; see chapter 5.

17. The beginnings of "functional diagnosis" are associated particularly with Ottomar Rosenbach (1851–1907). The best account of this movement in English is found in Faber, *Nosography.*

18. In a dye excretion test, a nontoxic dye is injected into the bloodstream, and its rate of appearance in the urine quantified. Administering a quantified amount of urea and assessing how quickly and fully the kidneys can excrete it was another assay once used (urea in the amount given was not toxic).

19. For "functional diagnosis" applied to the kidneys, see Faber, *Nosography,* 137–44; and Gabriel Richet, "Edema and Uremia from 1827 to 1905: The First Faltering Steps of Renal Pathophysiology," *Kidney International* 43 (1993): 1385–96.

20. For Addis and his contributions, see Steven J. Peitzman, "Thomas Addis (1881–1949): Mixing Patients, Rates, and Politics," *Kidney International* 37 (1990): 833–40.

21. The use of creatinine as a "marker" of glomerular filtration was developed largely by the Danish physiologist Poul Brandt Rehberg (1895–1985); see Carl W. Gottschalk, Robert W. Berliner, and Gerhard H. Giebisch, eds., *Renal Physiology: People and Ideas* (Bethesda, Md.: American Physiological Society, 1987), 42–43, 81–82, 166–67.

22. One million nephrons per human kidney has been the traditional teaching, but recent studies suggest a smaller, and more variable, number.

23. For the history of the low-protein diet in treating kidney disease, see: Allan Wasserstein, "Changing Patterns of Medical Practice: Protein Restriction for Chronic Renal Failure," *Annals of Internal Medicine* 119 (1993): 79–85; Joel Kopple, "History of Dietary Protein Therapy for the Treatment of Chronic Renal Disease from the Mid 1800s until the 1950s," *American Journal of Nephrology* 22 (2002): 278–83.

24. Thomas Addis, "Theory and Practice in the Dietetic Treatment of Glomerular Nephritis," *Journal of the American Dietetic Association* 16 (1940): 306–12, quote on pp. 311–12. Addis summarized his life's work on kidney disease, in the laboratory and clinic, in a remarkable book, *Glomerular Nephritis: Diagnosis and Treatment* (New York: McMillan, 1948).

25. Donald D. Van Slyke et al., "Observations on the Courses of Different Types of Bright's Disease, and on the Resultant Changes in Renal Anatomy," *Medicine* 9 (1930): 257–392. Van Slyke was known as a modest individual, generous to his students. The versatile "Van Slyke apparatus" allowed "gasometric" determination of carbon dioxide in the blood, urea in blood or urine, and other substances.

26. Robert Platt, *Nephritis and Allied Diseases: Their Pathogeny and Treatment* (London: Oxford University Press, 1934).

27. See Steven J. Peitzman, "Nephrology in America from Thomas Addis to the Artificial Kidney," in Russell C. Maulitz and Diana E. Long, eds., *Grand Rounds: One Hundred Years of Internal Medicine in America* (Philadelphia: University of Pennsylvania Press, 1988), 211–41 (an earlier version appeared as "Nephrology in the United States from Osler to the Artificial Kidney," *Annals of Internal Medicine* 105 [1986]: 937–46); Herbert Chasis and William Goldring, eds., *Homer William Smith, Sc. D.: His Scientific & Literary Achievements* (New York: New York University Press, 1965). Smith wrote one of the earliest comprehensive textbooks of renal physiology and disease, *The Kidney: Structure and Function in Health and Disease* (New York: Oxford University Press, 1951), which was known for many years among English-speaking renal specialists as "the bible." Its subtitle aptly indicates the themes of this chapter.

28. And of course, by the late twentieth century, both kidney function and disease had entered the realm of investigation at the molecular and genetic level.

29. Steven J. Peitzman, "Nephrology in America," 213.

30. This section is based on the following sources: Thomas Hager, *The Life of Linus Pauling* (New York: Simon and Schuster, 1995), 252–56; Linus Pauling, "Statement by a Former Patient, L.P.," in Kevin V. Lemley and Linus Pauling, "Thomas Addis July 27, 1881–June 4, 1949," *Biographical Memoirs of the National Academy of Sciences* 63 (1994): 23–24; files of correspondence about Pauling's kidney disease,

mostly between Thomas Addis and Ava Helen Pauling, but containing copies of other letters as well, in the Ava Helen and Linus Pauling Papers, Box 3, Special Collections, Oregon State University Libraries (copies kindly provided to the author, courtesy of the Pauling Papers; the author is grateful for the help of archivist Erika Castaño). The initial findings when Pauling was in New York are in Alfred E. Cohn to Addis, March 10, 1941. The removal of Dr. Pauling's teeth and his symptoms at home are from a letter of his local physician, Edwin McMillan, to Addis, March 21, 1941. Pauling has written about his kidney disorder and care by Thomas Addis, and it is described in the several published biographies, so no clinical confidentiality is being violated by the discussion in this book.

31. Some of her notebooks are preserved in the Pauling Papers.

32. Ava Helen Pauling to Addis, May 20, 1941, Pauling Papers.

33. Ava Helen Pauling to Addis, July 1, 1941, Pauling Papers.

34. Ava Helen Pauling to Addis, May 20, 1941, Pauling Papers.

35. McMillan to Addis, May 26, 1941, Pauling Papers.

36. Linus Pauling to Addis, June 19, 1941, Pauling Papers.

37. Linus Pauling Research Notebooks, Book 17, p. 15, June 1941, Pauling Papers, online at http://osulibrary.oregonstate.edu/specialcollections/rnb/17/17-015.html.

38. See Peitzman, "Thomas Addis."

39. Ava Helen Pauling to Addis, July 9, 1941; Addis to Ava Helen Pauling, October 7, 1941, Pauling Papers.

40. Addis to Linus Pauling, November 18, 1941, Pauling Papers.

41. Addis to Ava Helen Pauling, July 9, 1941, Pauling Papers.

42. Addis, *Glomerular Nephritis,* 311.

43. Case notes of P.H., Addis Papers, Library of Stanford University School of Medicine.

44. Addis to Ava Helen Pauling, September 13, 1943, Pauling Papers.

45. From his address "Doctor and Nurse," in *Aequanimitas: With Other Addresses to Medical Students, Nurses and Practitioners of Medicine,* 3rd ed. (Philadelphia: Blakiston, repr. 1932), 19. For other statements by Osler on the value of work, consult Mark Silverman, T. Jock Murray, and Charles S. Bryan, eds., *The Quotable Osler* (Philadelphia: The American College of Physicians, 2003); e.g., "Steady work . . . gives a man a sane outlook on the world" (p. 33).

46. Pamela Bright, *Dr. Richard Bright (1789–1858)* (London: Bodley Head, 1983).

47. Silas Weir Mitchell, *Doctor and Patient* (Philadelphia: Lippincott, 1900), 70.

48. Sheila M. Rothman, *Living in the Shadow of Death: Tuberculosis and the Social Experience of Illness in American History* (Baltimore: Johns Hopkins University Press, 1994), 26–44.

49. Pauling, "Statement by a Former Patient," 23. It seems likely that his long period of diet therapy under Addis, which included specified vitamin supplements, stimulated Pauling's later interest in preventive nutrition and vitamin C.

50. Nestor M. Pakasa and Ernest K. Sumlaili, "The Nephrotic Syndrome in the Democratic Republic of Congo," *New England Journal of Medicine* 354 (2006): 1085–86.

Chapter 5. Renal Shutdown, a Needle, and the End of Bright's Disease

1. Addis had also trained few disciples to keep his ideas alive, preferring his stable and familiar "group." His very left-leaning politics made association with Addis risky into the 1940s.

2. Alfred Fishman, Irving Kroop, Henry Leiter, and Abraham Hyman, "Experience with the Kolff Artificial Kidney," *American Journal of Medicine* 7 (1949): 15–34. The case narrative summarized here is on pp. 16–20.

3. The Royal Society of London for the Improvement of Natural Knowledge, usually known simply as the Royal Society, was chartered in 1663 and became the organizational framework for those engaged in the new forms of experimental investigation. Members included Robert Boyle, Robert Hooke, Isaac Newton, Christopher Wren, and many physicians.

4. The author was Mary Jane Ward, and the book is considered probably autobiographical. The film featured Olivia de Havilland.

5. For Gordon Murray's role in early hemodialysis, see J. Stewart Cameron, *A History of the Treatment of Renal Failure by Dialysis* (London: Oxford University Press, 2002), 80–87. A biography of Murray is Shelley McKellar, *Surgical Limits: The Life of Gordon Murray* (Toronto: University of Toronto Press, 2003).

6. Fishman, Kroop, Leiter, and Hyman, "Experience with the Kolff Artificial Kidney," 21.

7. Roy C. Swann and John P. Merrill, "The Clinical Course of Acute Renal Failure," *Medicine* 32 (1953): 215–92, quote on p. 216.

8. See Claus Brun, *Acute Anuria* (Copenhagen: Munksgaard, 1954), 11–24.

9. This type of acute renal failure has to be distinguished clinically from a sudden mechanical obstruction to urine flow, as can rarely occur with a stone, from certain forms of prostatic disease, and in other circumstances.

10. The hazards of the artificial kidney included the need for anticoagulation with heparin to prevent blood from clotting within the membrane tubing, and the potential for instability of the blood pressure.

11. For this debate in the United States, see Steven J. Peitzman, "Science, Inventors, and the Introduction of the Artificial Kidney in the United States," *Seminars in Dialysis* 9 (1996): 276–81.

12. For the "bichloride kidney," see Herman Elwyn, *Nephritis* (New York: Macmillan, 1926), 227–40; Arthur M. Fishberg, *Hypertension and Nephritis* (Philadelphia: Lea & Febiger, 1930), 250–56. For the history of mercuric chloride as a poison and agent of suicide, see Leonard J. Goldwater, *Mercury: A History of Quicksilver* (Baltimore: York Press, 1972), 165–68.

13. For the history of the sulfonamides, see Richard M. Weinshilboum, "The Therapeutic Revolution," *Clinical Pharmacology and Therapeutics* 42 (1987): 481–84; F. Hawling and J. Stewart Lawrence, *The Sulphonamides* (New York: Grune and Stratton, 1951), 1–8.

14. Eric Bywaters and Desmond Beall, "Crush Injuries with Impairment of Renal Function," *British Medical Journal* 1 (1941): 427–32, quote on p. 427.

15. Representative early articles and books on acute renal failure include Swann

and Merrill, "The Clinical Course of Acute Renal Failure"; John T. MacLean, *Acute Renal Failure Including the Use of the Artificial Kidney* (Springfield, Ill.: Charles C. Thomas, 1952); Claus Brun, *Acute Anuria;* Arthur Grollman, *Acute Renal Failure* (Springfield, Ill.: Charles C. Thomas, 1954); and John P. Merrill, *The Treatment of Acute Renal Failure* (New York: Grune and Stratton, 1955). The number of publications on acute renal failure increased sharply beginning in the late 1940s.

16. Acute renal failure of the myoglobinuric, or "crush injury," type is, however, still encountered, particularly following earthquakes. For the spectrum of causes of acute renal failure in the late twentieth and early twenty-first centuries, see Norbert Lameire et al., "The Changing Epidemiology of Acute Renal Failure," *Nature Clinical Practice Nephrology* 2 (2006): 364–77.

17. Paul M. Palevsky, "Acute Renal Failure," *NephSAP Nephrology Self-Assessment Program* 3 (2004): 252–59 (published by the American Society of Nephrology).

18. Steven J. Peitzman, "Richard Bright and Mercury as the Cause and Cure of Nephritis," *Bulletin of the History of Medicine* 52 (1978): 419–34.

19. John Chadwick and W. N. Mann, *The Medical Works of Hippocrates* (Oxford: Blackwell, 1950), 149.

20. For the history of organized nephrology in the United Kingdom, see J. Stewart Cameron, *First Half Century of the Renal Association,* 1959–2000, published as a pamphlet in 2000, and also available on the Association's Web site, www.renal.org. For a short overview of the history of nephrology as a specialty in the United States, see Steven J. Peitzman, "Nephrology in America from Thomas Addis to the Artificial Kidney," in Russell C. Maulitz and Diana E. Long, eds., *Grand Rounds: One Hundred Years of Internal Medicine in America* (Philadelphia: University of Pennsylvania Press, 1988), 211–41 (an earlier version appeared as "Nephrology in the United States from Osler to the Artificial Kidney," *Annals of Internal Medicine* 105 [1986]: 937–46).

21. E.g., hemolytic-uremic syndrome, thrombotic thrombocytopenic purpura, Goodpasture's syndrome, Wegener's granulomatosis, drug-induced acute interstitial nephritis.

22. For the early history of dialysis for acute renal failure, see Cameron, *History of the Treatment,* 121–56; Patrick T. McBride, *Genesis of the Artificial Kidney* (n.p.: Baxter Healthcare, 1987), 19–32; and Peitzman, "Science, Inventors, and the Introduction of the Artificial Kidney." The physicians associated with early dialysis care in Washington, D.C., and Korea include Paul Doolan, George Schreiner, and Paul Teschan (who supervised the treatments at the field hospital).

23. Another technique, peritoneal dialysis, also found extensive use in dealing with acute renal failure, especially in clinical settings in which maintaining the expertise to conduct hemodialysis was not possible. In peritoneal dialysis, still in use for acute and chronic disease, physiologically balanced sterile fluid is entered into the abdominal cavity through an implanted catheter. The fluid draws solutes from the blood using the capillaries of the abdominal mesentery as the effective separating membrane. The fluid is then drained out by gravity. It is also possible to remove excess bodily fluids with this technique, which requires no complex machinery. Peritoneal dialysis is, however, less effective in a unit of time than hemodialysis, and

sometimes a disease process within the abdomen precludes its use in a very sick individual.

24. Poul Iversen and Claus Brun, "Aspiration Biopsy of the Kidney," *American Journal of Medicine* 11 (1951): 324–30, quote from p. 324. Iversen had earlier performed percutaneous biopsy of the liver. The phrase "utero-placental damage" refers to another occasional source of acute renal failure, namely, certain obstetrical complications associated with severe bleeding and sometimes infection. For the history of renal biopsy, see: Robert M. Kark, "The Development of Percutaneous Renal Biopsy in Man," *American Journal of Kidney Diseases* 16 (1990): 585–89; idem, "Renal Biopsy and the Modern Era," in J. Stewart Cameron and Richard J. Glassock, eds., *The Nephrotic Syndrome* (New York: Dekker, 1988), 57–86; J. Stewart Cameron and J. Hicks, "The Introduction of Renal Biopsy into Nephrology from 1901 to 1961: A Paradigm of the Forming of Nephrology by Technology," *American Journal of Nephrology* 17 (1997): 346–58. Nils Alwall (1906–1986), an enormously versatile and accomplished Swedish pioneer of nephrology, had performed some biopsies in the early 1940s but did not report them until later.

25. Alvin E. Parrish and John Howe, "Kidney Biopsy: A Review of One Hundred Successful Needle Biopsies," *Archives of Internal Medicine* 96 (1955): 712–16. Nephrosclerosis refers to the renal histological appearance showing alterations dominantly in the small arterial blood vessels, along with destruction of glomeruli and fibrotic scarring. This appearance is associated with long-standing high blood pressure in the patient.

26. These articles appeared in *Lancet, New England Journal of Medicine, American Journal of Medicine,* and *Journal of Clinical Investigation.* A bibliography is available in Kark's chapter on biopsy in Cameron and Glassock, *The Nephrotic Syndrome.*

27. Renal biopsy also revealed from time to time the appearance of amyloidosis, the "lardaceous kidney" of the nineteenth century. It also added much information about acute poststreptococcal glomerulonephritis and other disorders not discussed here.

28. "The art consists in three things—the disease, the patient, and the physician. The physician is the servant of the art, and the patient must combat the disease along with the physician" (*Of the Epidemics*).

Chapter 6. Inventing Chronic Dialysis

1. United States Renal Data System, "Excerpts from the United States Renal Data System 2004 Annual Data Report" (also referred to as the 2005 report in some of the page headings), *American Journal of Kidney Diseases* 45, suppl. 1 (2005): S1–S280, 20.

2. Lee Foster, "Man and Machine: Life without Kidneys," *Hastings Center Report* 6 (1976): 5–8. Mr. Foster at the time was assistant travel editor for the *New York Times.*

3. Connie Jones, ed., *Even in Heaven They Don't Sing All the Time: Experiences of Kidney Patients and Their Families* (Atlanta: National Kidney Foundation of Georgia, 1984), 21, 41–43. This small volume contains a collection of moving and fascinating narratives of chronic dialysis recipients from one clinic.

4. Harry S. Abram, "Survival by Machine: The Psychological Stress of Chronic Hemodialysis," *Psychiatry in Medicine* 1 (1972): 37–51; quotation from p. 44.

5. "Extending Life or Prolonging Death? The Dialysis Dilemma," *New York Times,* March 23, 1986.

6. John P. Merrill, *The Treatment of Renal Failure* (New York City: Grune and Stratton, 1955), 193–94. For early use of dialysis in chronic patients, see ibid., 190–94; Willem J. Kolff, "Artificial Kidney: Treatment of Acute and Chronic Uremia," *Cleveland Clinic Quarterly* 17 (1950): 216–28; Donna K. McCurdy and Lewis W. Bluemle, "The Current Status of Hemodialysis," *Medical Clinics of North America* 47 (1963): 1043–56. For a biography of Merrill, see Nancy Boucot Cummings, "John Putnam Merrill: An Appreciation," *Artificial Organs* 11 (1987): 438–41.

7. There exists an enormous historical literature on the beginnings of chronic dialysis, e.g.: Richard Rettig, *Health Care Technology: Lessons Learned from the End-Stage Renal Disease Experience* (Santa Monica, Calif.: Rand Corporation, 1976); Renée C. Fox and Judith P. Swazey, *The Courage to Fail: A Social View of Organ Transplantation and Dialysis,* 2nd ed. (Chicago: University of Chicago Press, 1978); Belding Scribner, "A Personalized History of Chronic Hemodialysis," *American Journal of Kidney Diseases* 16 (1990): 511–19; Steven J. Peitzman, "Chronic Dialysis and Dialysis Doctors in the United States: A Nephrologist-Historian's Perspective," *Seminars in Dialysis* 14 (2001): 200–208; J. Stewart Cameron, *A History of the Treatment of Renal Failure by Dialysis* (London: Oxford University Press, 2002), 187–93.

8. Fox and Swazey, *Courage to Fail,* 202. The names of Scribner's patients have appeared widely in print already, and so are used here without concern for confidentiality.

9. Scribner's initial publications on the shunt and chronic dialysis are: Wayne Quinton, David Dillard, and Belding Scribner, "Cannulation of Blood Vessels for Prolonged Hemodialysis," *Transactions of the American Society for Artificial Internal Organs* 6 (1960): 104–13, and Scribner et al., "The Treatment of Chronic Uremia by Means of Intermittent Hemodialysis: A Preliminary Report," *Transactions of the American Society for Artificial Internal Organs* 6 (1960): 114–22.

10. Fox and Swazey, *Courage to Fail,* 206. Scribner understood that his program could not indefinitely consume hospital funds and space. The university nonetheless maintained a dialysis unit for acute treatments, with an emphasis on research.

11. Judith S. Jacobson, *The Greatest Good: A History of the John A. Hartford Foundation* (n.p.: The Hartford Foundation, 1984), 55. Hartford support for renal dialysis and transplantation is discussed on pp. 35–62.

12. For the life and work of Belding Scribner, see the author's entry in William Bynum and Helen Bynum, eds., *Dictionary of Medical Biography* (Westport, Conn.: Greenwood Press, 2006).

13. For example, Norman Levinsky, a Boston nephrologist whose research concerned renal sodium handling, cautiously advised in a review published by the influential *New England Journal of Medicine* in 1964 that "both chronic dialysis and transplantation, except between identical twins, are properly considered clinical experiments rather than established modes of treatment at this time." Levinsky, "Management of Chronic Renal Failure. Part 2," *New England Journal of Medicine* 271

(1964): 458–63, quote at p. 463. In this review Levinsky offers what surely must be one of the most optimistic suggestions ever provided in the realm of medical interviewing: "Every patient with irreversible renal failure should be questioned about the existence of an identical twin" (p. 462).

14. See Keatha K. Krueger, ed., *Proceedings of Annual Contractors' Conference on the Artificial Kidney* (Bethesda, Md.: Public Health Service, National Institutes of Health, 1969), 13; Rettig, *Health Care Technology,* 16–17. The U.S. National Institutes of Health in 1965 created the Artificial Kidney–Chronic Uremia Program within the National Institute of Arthritis and Metabolic Diseases to award research contracts aimed at technical improvement in dialysis.

15. United States Kidney Disease Control Program, *Kidney Disease Services, Facilities, and Programs in the United States* (Arlington, Va.: Government Printing Office, 1969); Cameron, *History of the Treatment,* 220.

16. See Cameron, *History of the Treatment,* 193–94; James Cimino and Michael Brescia, "The Early Development of the Arteriovenous Fistula Needle Technique for Hemodialysis," *American Society for Artificial Internal Organs Journal* 40 (1994): 923–27.

17. See Fox and Swazey, *Courage to Fail,* 226–65. Some sources state that the committee included only laypersons, whereas others suggest physicians also participated.

18. The most sharp and shrill criticism is found in David Sanders and Jesse Dukeminier, "Medical Advance and Legal Lag: Hemodialysis and Kidney Transplantation," *UCLA Law Review* 15 (1968): 357–413.

19. Carl Gottschalk, *Report of the Committee on Chronic Kidney Disease* (n.p., 1967). This report was commissioned by the U.S. Bureau of Budget in order to learn about the likely expenses that would be entailed by the growth of chronic dialysis, and the desirability of establishing a federal payment program. Carl Gottschalk (1922–1997) was a distinguished nephrologist and renal physiologist whose career was mainly at the University of North Carolina in Chapel Hill. He was uniformly respected, and he wasn't personally involved in hemodialysis or advocacy for it in its early years.

20. Ibid., 85–99.

21. Judith Mausner et al., "An Area Wide Survey of Treated End-Stage Renal Disease," *American Journal of Public Health* 68 (1978): 166–97; Steven J. Rosansky and Paul W. Eggers, "Trends in the US End-Stage Renal Disease Population: 1973–1983," *American Journal of Kidney Diseases* 9 (1987): 91–97.

22. The cost of dialysis in a chronic unit for one year in the mid-1960s was estimated to be about $14,000, a figure equal to the annual salary for many sorts of service jobs at that time. The phrase "needless deaths" was repeated often in the debates over funding chronic dialysis. For example, it was publicly used by Senator Vance Hartke of Indiana in comments added to a Senate Finance Committee report of September 1972 (quoted in Richard Rettig, "Origins of the Medicare Kidney Disease Entitlement: The Social Security Amendments of 1972," in Kathi E. Hanna, ed., *Biomedical Politics* [Washington: Institute of Medicine and National Academy Press, 1981], 192).

23. A great deal has been written about the Medicare amendment for chronic kidney disease. The best sources include Fox and Swazey, *Courage to Fail*, 345–56; David J. Rothman, *Beginnings Count: The Technological Imperative in American Health Care* (New York: Oxford University Press, 1997), 94–109; Rettig, "Origins"; George Schreiner, "How End-Stage Renal Disease (ESRD)–Medicare Developed," *Seminars in Nephrology* 17 (1997): 152–59.

24. Medicare coverage was expanded from those over sixty-five years old to the disabled by another section of the same 1972 amendments.

25. The dollar figures are from United States Renal Data System, "Excerpts," 20.

26. For the emergence of National Medical Care, Inc., the first commercial dialysis network, see: Fox and Swazey, *Courage to Fail*, 363–65; Alonzo Plough, *Borrowed Time: Artificial Organs and the Politics of Extending Lives* (Philadelphia: Temple University Press, 1986), 155–73; Gina Bari Kolata, "N.M.C. Thrives Selling Dialysis," *Science* 208 (1980): 379–82.

27. Arnold Relman, "The New Medical-Industrial Complex," *New England Journal of Medicine* 303 (1980): 963–70. Relman, a nephrologist, was chairman of medicine at the University of Pennsylvania School of Medicine before assuming editorship of the *New England Journal of Medicine*.

28. The literature carrying on this debate is of course voluminous. See, in addition to items already cited: John K. Inglehart, "Funding the End-Stage Renal-Disease Program," *New England Journal of Medicine* 306 (1982): 492–96; Edmund G. Lowrie and Constantine L. Hampers, "Medicare's End-Stage Renal Disease Program: Historical and Policy Considerations," in Robert G. Narins, ed., *Controversies in Nephrology and Hypertension* (New York: Churchill Livingstone, 1984), 5-23; Allan Hull, "The Legislative and Regulatory Process in the End-Stage Renal Disease (ESRD) Program, 1973 through 1997," *Seminars in Nephrology* 17 (1997): 160–69.

29. For a synopsis of the basic data and issues, see Alan R. Hull and Tom F. Parker, "Introduction and Summary: Proceedings from the Morbidity, Mortality and Prescription of Dialysis Symposium, Dallas, TX, September 15 to 17, 1989," *American Journal of Kidney Diseases* 15 (1990): 375–83. For several perspectives on these findings and their basis, see Eli A. Friedman, "End-Stage Renal Disease Therapy: An American Success Story," *Journal of the American Medical Association* 275 (1996): 1118-22; Richard Rettig, "The Social Contract and the Treatment of Permanent Kidney Failure," *Journal of the American Medical Association* 275 (1996): 1123-28; J. Michael Lazarus and Allen R. Nissenson, eds., "Proceedings from Comprehensive Management of Dialysis Patients in the 1990s," published as supplement 1 of *American Journal of Kidney Diseases* 20 (July 1992).

30. See Allen R. Nissenson, "Morbidity and Mortality of United States Dialysis Patients—The Legacy of Inadequate Nephrologist Training?" *Seminars in Dialysis* 5 (1992): 277–78.

31. These included the development of better dialyzing membranes and the utilization of higher flow rates for blood entering the filter and for the dialyzing fluid, which carries off the waste substances that have diffused across the filter.

32. See Wolfgang Schivelbusch, *The Railway Journey: The Industrialization of*

Time and Space in the 19th Century (Berkeley: University of California Press, 1986), a translation of *Geschichte der Eisenbahnreise,* published in 1977; English translation originally published 1979), esp. 113-23.

33. William N. McClellan, "The Epidemic of End-Stage Renal Disease in the United States: A Public Health Perspective on ESRD Prevention," *AKF Nephrology Newsletter* 10 (1993): 29–40.

34. Cameron, *History of the Treatment,* 317–23.

35. Peitzman, "Chronic Dialysis and Dialysis Doctors." Though not widely placed in print, another concern of some leaders of American nephrology was that the proliferation of chronic dialysis might reduce expenditures for research, as well as consume excessive amounts of time within academic nephrology divisions and training programs.

36. Robert Steinbrook, "Medicare and Erythropoietin," *New England Journal of Medicine* 356 (2007): 4–6.

Chapter 7. Coupled to the Artificial Kidney

1. I came upon this pamphlet (Public Health Service Publication no. 1810) at the Library of the College of Physicians of Philadelphia, where so much of my research took place, but have never been able to establish the exact objective of its publication. It is an extraordinary pictorial artifact.

2. The phrase was applied to Scribner's patients by an early figure in hemodialysis in Philadelphia (and later president of Jefferson Medical College), Lewis Bluemle, in "Treatment at Home: Crucial Test for Hemodialysis," *Medical World News,* November 6, 1964, 95–102, quote on p. 100.

3. Home hemodialysis was also less expensive than that done in a center.

4. Jennifer Castillo, "A View from the La-Z-Boy Chair," *Advances in Renal Replacement Therapy* 9 (2002): 224-25.

5. One woman, Lori Hartwell, a veteran of hemodialysis, the alternative modality peritoneal dialysis, and three kidney transplants, has become a successful motivational speaker and author (her book is *Chronically Happy: Joyful Living in Spite of Chronic Illness*). When he was "Britain's longest surviving dialysis patient," Brian Tocher wrote and published his life story, *Chronic Kidney Failure—Treatment & Diet.*

6. In chronic peritoneal dialysis, a plastic catheter is surgically placed through the abdominal wall into the abdominal cavity, allowing the repeated introduction and drainage of a physiological solution. When this solution "dwells" in the abdominal cavity, urea, creatinine, potassium, and other solutes to be removed diffuse into it across the capillary and peritoneal membranes. One either does four or five exchanges during the day (at home, work, etc.) or utilizes a "cycler" device that carries out a series of exchanges overnight, during sleep. Peritoneal dialysis allows more flexibility and independence and avoids the risk of introducing infection into the bloodstream that occurs with hemodialysis. However, abdominal infection can occur with peritoneal dialysis, and its effectiveness is inadequate for very large persons. Sometimes it cannot be done if a person has had past abdominal surgery.

7. Some had polycystic kidney disease, an inherited disorder that can cause renal failure by midadult life.

8. The pathologic alteration in the glomerulus is also referred to as intercapillary glomerulosclerosis or Kimmelstiel-Wilson Disease after the American physician Paul Kimmelstiel and British physician Clifford Wilson, who, working together, published an important paper on the subject in 1936. For the history of diabetic renal disease, see J. Stewart Cameron, *A History of the Treatment of Renal Failure by Dialysis* (Oxford: Oxford University Press, 2002), 293–99; Garabed Eknoyan and Judit Nagy, "A History of Diabetes Mellitus or How a Disease of the Kidneys Evolved into a Kidney Disease," *Advances in Chronic Kidney Disease* 12 (2005): 223-29.

9. For demographics of dialysis in the United States, see United States Renal Data System, "Excerpts from the United States Renal Data System 2004 Annual Data Report" (also referred to as the 2005 report in some of the page headings), *American Journal of Kidney Diseases* 45, suppl. 1 (2005): S1–S280. The trends toward many more older patients and patients with diabetic renal disease was well evident by the late 1970s; see Steven J. Rosansky and Paul W. Eggers, "Trends in the US End-Stage Renal Disease Population: 1973–1983," *American Journal of Kidney Diseases* 9 (1987): 91–97.

10. William F. Owen, Jr., "Racial Differences in Incidence, Outcome, and Quality of Life for African-Americans on Hemodialysis," *Blood Purification* 14 (1996): 278–85.

11. This was the first NIH clinical trial centered on a minority group, and its creation at first attracted some controversy, though I know of little or none that ensued later. Its initial results, which showed the superiority of one class of antihypertensive medication in slowing the worsening of hypertensive renal disease among blacks, appeared in Lawrence Y. Agodoa et al., "Effect of Ramipril vs. Amlodipine on Renal Outcomes in Hypertensive Nephrosclerosis: A Randomized Control Trial," *Journal of the American Medical Association* 285 (2001): 2719-28.

12. The medical and related literature on the disproportionate amount of kidney disease among persons of color (and other minority groups) is now vast. It mainly addresses possible biological and socioeconomic explanations for the disparity but also issues of access to care. One of the first important papers to identify the disparity was Stephen G. Rostand et al., "Racial Differences in the Incidence of Treatment for End-Stage Renal Disease," *New England Journal of Medicine* 306 (1982): 1276–79. Other recent (as this is written) reviews and key articles include: K. C. Norris and Lawrence Agodoa, "Unraveling the Racial Disparities with Kidney Disease," *Kidney International* 68 (2005): 1364–65; Michelle Tarver-Carr et al., "Excess Risk of Chronic Renal Disease among African-American versus White Subjects in the United States: A Population-Based Study of Potential Explanatory Factors," *Journal of the American Society of Nephrology* 13 (2002): 2363–70; Carlton Young and Robert Gaston, "Renal Transplantation in Black Americans," *New England Journal of Medicine* 343 (2000): 1545–52; Saulo Klahr, "Transforming Growth Factor Beta 1 and Renal Disease in African Americans," *Kidney International* 53 (1998): 792–93; Eric W. Young et al., "Socioeconomic Status and End-Stage Renal Disease in the United States," *Kidney International* 45 (1994): 907–11; Richard Sherman et al., "Racial Differences in the Delivery of Hemodialysis," *American Journal of Kidney Diseases* 21 (1993): 632–34; Frederick L. Brancati et al., "The Excess Incidence of Diabetic End-

Stage Renal Disease among Blacks," *Journal of the American Medical Association* 268 (1992): 3079–84; Stephen G. Rostand, "Hypertension and Renal Disease in Blacks: Role of Genetic and/or Environmental Factors?" *Advances in Nephrology* 21 (1992): 99–116; Rollington Ferguson, "End-Stage Renal Disease and Race: An Overview and Perspective," *Journal of the National Medical Association* 83 (1991): 794–98. A supplement to the February 2003 issue of the journal *Kidney International,* "Renal Disease in Racial and Ethnic Minority Groups," comprises a wide range of articles (vol. 63, suppl. 83). An interesting commentary, though not focusing on renal disease, is Newton G. Osborne and Marvin D. Feit, "The Use of Race in Medical Research," *Journal of the American Medical Association* 267 (1992): 275–79.

13. For some evocation of this experience, see Laurie Kaye Abraham, *Mama Might Be Better Off Dead: The Failure of Health Care in Urban America* (Chicago: University of Chicago Press, 1993), 25–43. Chapter 7, however, does not express the notion of an entirely failed health care system.

14. My conclusions about awareness of kidney disease as reflected in African-American periodicals are based on a review of the *Reader's Guide to Periodic Literature* from 1990 through 1994, and a search of the "Multicultural" database of *Proquest* through 2005. These and other tasks were skillfully carried out for me by Corinna Schlombs, then a graduate student in the Department of the History and Sociology of Science of the University of Pennsylvania. One of very few articles identified is "Why Blacks Suffer More from Kidney Disease," in *Jet,* April 21, 1997.

15. For the ramifications of an "African-American Disease," see Keith Wailoo's masterful *Dying in the City of the Blues: Sickle Cell Anemia and the Politics of Race and Health* (Chapel Hill: University of North Carolina Press, 2001).

16. Connie Jones, *Even in Heaven They Don't Sing All the Time: Experiences of Kidney Patients and Their Families* (Atlanta: National Kidney Foundation of Georgia, 1984), 34.

17. Penelope Ellison, "Holding It Together: Managing Lives around Kidney Disease," *About . . . Time* 23 (1995): 22.

18. Withdrawal from dialysis has been studied most boldly and carefully by nephrologist Carl Kjellstrand; see, e.g., his article (with coauthors) "Dialysis Discontinuation and Palliative Care," *American Journal of Kidney Diseases* 36 (2000): 140–44.

19. Melanie K. Landsman, "The Patient with Chronic Renal Failure: A Marginal Man," *Annals of Internal Medicine* 82 (1975): 268–70.

20. Peter Lundin, "A Personal Experience of Twenty-Four Years of Dialysis," *Transplantation Proceedings* 22 (1990): 957–58, quote on p. 957.

21. Lee Foster, "Man and Machine: Life without Kidneys," *Hastings Center Reports* 6 (1976): 5–8, quote on p. 8.

22. Chase Patterson Kimball and Richard Allen Famularo, "The Experience of Hemodialysis and Renal Transplantation," *General Hospital Psychiatry* 2 (1980): 70–80, quote on p. 72.

23. Foster, "Man and Machine," 7.

24. H. Katherine O'Neill and Russell E. Glasgow, "Patient Perceptions of the Hemodialysis Regimen," *Loss, Grief and Care* 5 (1991): 167–76.

25. Steven D. Weisbord et al., "Prevalence, Severity, and Importance of Physical and Emotional Symptoms in Chronic Hemodialysis Patients," *Journal of the American Society of Nephrology* 16 (2005): 2487–94. This paper reported on patients at three dialysis units in the Pittsburgh, Pennsylvania, region. Sleep problems were also common.

26. For an overview of the entry of epoetin-alpha into the practice of chronic dialysis, see Cameron, *History of the Treatment,* 287–93.

27. Information about Amgen is from the "Company History" section of its Internet site, www.amgen.com, accessed May 29, 2006.

28. Ernst P. Boas, *The Unseen Plague: Chronic Disease* (New York: J. J. Augustin, 1940), 22. Boas certainly insisted on the importance of treating pain. See also the chapter "The Discovery of Chronic Disease" in Gerald N. Grob, *The Deadly Truth: A History of Disease in America* (Cambridge, Mass.: Harvard University Press, 2002).

29. Though I have not sought specific evidence, I consider it entirely likely that Addis knew Boas and had read *The Unseen Plague.*

30. One such supporter, Senator Vance Hartke, asserted during the deliberation over dialysis in 1972 that 60 percent of patients would be able to return to work with "retraining," and 40 percent directly; cited in Richard A. Rettig, "The Policy Debate on Patient Care Financing for Victims of End-Stage Renal Disease," *Law and Contemporary Problems* 40 (1976): 196-230, esp. 224.

31. There were many publications on vocational rehabilitation in the 1980s and into the 1990s. See, e.g., N. G. Kutner et al., "Employment Status and Ability to Work among Working-Age Chronic Dialysis Patients," *American Journal of Nephrology* 11 (1991): 334–40; K. King, "Vocational Rehabilitation in Maintenance Dialysis Patients," *Advances in Renal Replacement Therapy* 1 (1994): 229–39. Among the bleakest reports are those authored by senior nephrologist Eli Friedman and his colleagues at the Downstate Medical Center in a poor area of Brooklyn, e.g., "Pervasive Failed Rehabilitation in Center-Based Maintenance Hemodialysis Patients," *American Journal of Kidney Diseases* 23 (1994): 394–400.

32. The quotations are from, in order: Ariela Royer, *Life with Chronic Disease: Social and Psychological Dimensions* (Westport, Conn.: Praeger, 1998), 66; George Harper, "Home Hemodialysis: A Patient's Perspective," *Hemodialysis International* 1 (1997): 8–11, quote on p. 10; Castillo, "A View from the La-Z-Boy Chair," 225; Anonymous, "Haemodialysis," *Lancet* 2 (October 10, 1981): 800–801, quote on p. 800; Jones, *Even in Heaven,* 4.

33. Both quotes are from Richard Rettig and Norman Levinsky, eds., *Kidney Failure and the Federal Government* (Washington, D.C.: Institute of Medicine and the National Academy Press, 1991), 48. For the realities of work and getting by as experienced by some inner-city hemodialysis recipients, see Abraham, *Mama Might Be Better Off Dead,* 36–43.

34. Quotes from: Jones, *Even in Heaven,* 4; "The Numbers Keep Growing: African-Americans Living with Kidney Disease," *New Pittsburgh Courier,* May 27, 1995.

35. Of course, something of the sort can become the case for persons with other

kinds of chronic diseases, as they follow complicated medication schedules, perhaps follow a restricted diet or engage in physical therapy, and manage appointments with a primary physician and half a dozen or more consultants.

36. See, e.g., Nathan Levin, "Quality of Life and Hematocrit Level," *American Journal of Kidney Diseases* 20, suppl. 1 (1992): S16–S20.

37. See Edith T. Oberley et al., "Renal Rehabilitation: Obstacles, Progress, and Prospects for the Future," *American Journal of Kidney Diseases* 35, suppl. 1 (2000): S141–S147.

38. These examples are drawn from various published accounts and from my own earlier experience as a nephrologist with the Veterans Administration, when I was engaged in more care of persons on dialysis than I have been recently.

39. Quotes are from: Gillian Brunier, "Appraising and Monitoring a Life on Dialysis," *Canadian Association of Nephrology Nurses and Technicians Bulletin* (Summer 1990): 15–17, quote on p. 15; Jones, *Even in Heaven,* 7; Foster, "Man and Machine," 7; Ermine Saner, " 'I Can't Imagine Not Sharing My Life with This Machine': Patricia LeBlack May Be the Longest-Surviving Kidney Dialysis Patient in the World," *Guardian,* September 21, 2006, accessed online November 26, 2006, at www.guardian.co.uk/g2/story/0,,1877244,00.html.

40. For a brief look at self-control in American culture, or its lack, see Daniel Akst, "Who's in Charge Here?" *Wilson Quarterly* 30 (Summer 2006): 31–37.

41. Alonzo Plough, *Borrowed Time: Artificial Organs and the Politics of Extending Life* (Philadelphia: Temple University Press, 1986).

Chapter 8. The Gift of Life

1. Jason Diamos, "Mourning Comes Back: How Long Will He Stay?" *New York Times,* October 29, 2004.

2. Liz Robbins, "Mourning Has Taken the Road Less Traveled to the Finals," *New York Times,* June 4, 2006.

3. Mike Wise, "Mourning Returns, Tilting the Balance of Power," *New York Times,* March 28, 2001.

4. Of course, many persons on dialysis, especially younger ones, do work out and engage in sports, hiking, bicycling, etc.

5. Ortho Biotech Products, "NBA Star Alonzo Mourning Spreads the Word about Kidney Disease" (press release), June 28, 2005, accessed online June 3, 2006 at www.orthobiotech.com/050628.html.

6. Ibid.

7. "Alonzo Mourning's Comeback from Kidney Disease Makes Miami Heat Center an All-Star On and Off the Court," *Jet,* March 18, 2002, 48–51, quote from p. 48. Other coverage of Mourning's renal disease in *Jet* are found in the following issues: October 7, 2002; January 19, 2004; and for Sean Elliott, August 16, 1999.

8. Keith Wailoo, *Dying in the City of the Blues: Sickle Cell Anemia and the Politics of Race and Health* (Chapel Hill: University of North Carolina Press, 2001).

9. One might consider blood transfusion as a form of organ transplantation with priority over successful kidney grafting. For the general history of renal transplantation, see: Nicholas Tilney, *Transplant: From Myth to Reality* (New Haven, Conn.:

Yale University Press, 2003); Vassilios Papalois et al., "The History of Kidney Transplantation," in Nadey Hakim and Vassilios Papalois, eds., *History of Organ and Cell Transplantation* (London: Imperial College Press, 2003), 76–99; David Hamilton, "Reaching for the Impossible: The Quest for Tissue Replacement," in Leo C. Ginns et al., eds., *Transplantation* (Malden, Mass.: Blackwell Science, 1999), 1–19.

10. See Francis D. Moore, *Give and Take: The Development of Tissue Transplantation* (Philadelphia: Saunders, 1964), 13–15. There seems not to have been a report of this 1947 transplantation in the period soon after it was done.

11. Later accounts of this case state that she died five months later from hepatitis acquired from a blood transfusion given as part of the initial treatment of her severe illness.

12. Interview with George Thorn by Steven Peitzman, May 28, 1991 (transcript on deposit at the Countway Library of Harvard Medical School, Boston), 26-27; G. W. Thorn, "A 50th Anniversary Celebration," *Transplantation Proceedings* 13, suppl. 1 (1981): 24-28.

13. Tilney, *Transplant,* 49–50.

14. Shelley McKellar, *Surgical Limits: The Life of Gordon Murray* (Toronto: University of Toronto Press, 2003), 92–95; Vivian Charles McAlister, "Clinical Kidney Transplantation: A 50th Anniversary Review of the First Reported Series," *American Journal of Surgery* 190 (2005): 485–88.

15. David Hume et al., "Experiences with Renal Homotransplantation in the Human: Report of Nine Cases," *Journal of Clinical Investigation* 34 (1955): 327–82, quotation on p. 378. Later, the word "allograft" by consensus came into use to describe an organ transplanted from one person, or animal, to another. A "homograft" then would be an organ transplanted from one place in a human or animal to another place in the same human or animal, such as a skin graft in the case of burn injury.

16. For the history of the early transplants in twins, see: John P. Merrill et al., "Successful Homotransplantation of the Human Kidney between Identical Twins," *Journal of the American Medical Association* 160 (1956): 277–82; Joseph Murray et al., "Kidney Transplantation between Seven Pairs of Identical Twins," *Annals of Surgery* 148 (1958): 343–59; Tilney, *Transplant,* 60–67; Moore, *Give and Take,* 69–77.

17. See, e.g., Laura Johannes, "Delicate Surgery: In Kidney Quest, New Rules Boost Chances for Blacks," *Wall Street Journal,* June 18, 2004.

18. Cyclosporin became critical in the routinization of transplantation of hearts and livers.

19. There exists an abundance of literature on the ethical, sociological, and psychological aspects of organ transplantation. This literature includes two volumes by Renée C. Fox and Judith P. Swazey: *The Courage to Fail: A Social View of Organ Transplants and Dialysis,* 2nd ed. (Chicago: University of Chicago Press, 1978), and *Spare Parts: Organ Replacement in American Society* (New York: Oxford University Press, 1992). See also two anthologies: Stuart J. Youngner, Renée C. Fox, and Laurence J. O'Connell, eds., *Organ Transplantation: Meanings and Realities* (Madison, Wis.: University of Wisconsin Press, 1996), and James R. Rodrigue, ed., *Biopsychosocial Perspectives on Transplantation* (New York: Kluwer Academic / Plenum, 2001). I do not claim to have read all of these in entirety.

20. United States Renal Data System, "Excerpts from the United States Renal Data System 2004 Annual Data Report" (also referred to as the 2005 report in some of the page headings), *American Journal of Kidney Diseases* 45, suppl. 1 (2005): S1–S280; also available via www.usrds.org.

21. See U.S. Department of Health and Human Services, 2005 *Annual Report of the U.S. Organ Procurement and Transplantation Network and the Scientific Registry of Transplant Recipients* (Rockville, Md., 2005); also available at www.ustransplant.org.

22. These three quotations are from: Penelope Ellison, "Holding It Together: Managing Lives around Kidney Disease," *About . . . Time* 23 (1995): 22 (accessed online via ProQuest); "People Like You: Hear What Dialysis Patients Have to Say about Their Transplant Experiences," www.transplantlife.com (Astellas Pharma US, Inc.), accessed February 5, 2006; Al Sabatini, "A Tale of Two Kidneys," in "How the Patients See It," chap. 11 of the KT/DA (Kidney Transplantation/Dialysis Association) *Patient Handbook,* accessed online, July 5, 2006, at http://msl1.mit.edu/ESD10/kidneys/HndbkHTML/contents.htm. KT/DA is an organization centered in New England.

23. Debora Persichetti, "October," in National Kidney Foundation Web site, "Transplant Stories," www.kidney.org/transplantation/transAction/shareShowStory.cfm?storyID=118, accessed June 16, 2006. Such Web sites do tend to feature stories of endurance and success.

24. For one account of the recovery period after renal donation, see Martha McNeil Hamilton and Warren Brown, *Black and White and Red All Over* (New York: Public Affairs, 2002), 189–205. The laparoscopic removal of the donor kidney is, however, substantially less of an operation than the previous techniques, and its availability may be a factor in the increased willingness to donate.

25. The pamphlet is USPHS (United States Public Health Service) publication 1801. The copy I used is at the Library of the College of Physicians of Philadelphia. The phrase "miracle of modern medical technology" is on an initial, unnumbered page of introductory text. The reference to "difficulties, frustrations, inconveniences, and tensions" is on p. 16. The pamphlet lists no author, and I have been unable to learn anything of its genesis.

26. Numerous periodical and newspaper articles can be found using ProQuest, and online stories of transplantation by using the familiar search engines. One can enter, e.g., "kidney transplantation gift of life."

27. Emily Yellen, "A Teacher's Gift? Why, Most Certainly," *New York Times,* December 18, 1999.

28. Dianne Anderson, "A Brother's Love: When Crisis Hits Home," *Precinct Reporter* (San Bernardino) 31, 6 (1995): A-1.

29. Marie Black, "The True Meaning of 'Brotherly Love,'" *Call and Post* (Cleveland), June 12, 1997.

30. Kiran Randhawa, "Best Friend Saved My Life with Her Gift of a Kidney," *Evening Standard* (London), June 26, 2006.

31. Kathryn Wenner, "Sharing More Than a Corner of the Office," *American Journalism Review* 24 (2002): 12–13. For their remarkable, jointly told, full story, see Hamilton and Brown, *Black and White and Red All Over.*

32. See, e.g., Fox and Swazey, *Spare Parts,* 36–42.

33. "Local Organ Transplant Patient Mitchell Welch Is Grateful to Have Received His Kidney," *Sacramento Observer* 42, 29 (July 7–13, 2005): 7. In the case of deceased donor transplantation, instances in which either family members of the donor or the recipient have sought contact between the two parties have sometimes proved problematic, and some (not all) transplantation professionals discourage such interaction.

34. Quoted in Fox and Swazey, *Spare Parts,* 39.

35. I am grateful to Toby Appel, PhD, MSLS, for calling my attention to the Transplant Games, and for other suggestions regarding this chapter. These events are open to recipients of all organ transplants, not just kidneys.

36. Although I am not aware that previous writers about kidney transplantation have focused on stories in the popular press, I claim no originality for my commentary about transplantation and gift-giving. Among the earliest scholars to think carefully about these interactions were Renée C. Fox and Judith Swazey; see, e.g., *Spare Parts,* 31–48, and references in that volume to their earlier contributions.

37. See Wendy Doniger, "Transplanting Myths of Organ Transplants," in Youngner, Fox, and O'Connell, *Organ Transplantation,* 194–220.

Chapter 9. Progression and Renewal

1. Jason Diamos, "Mourning Comes Back: How Long Will He Stay?" *New York Times,* October 29, 2004; "Alonzo Mourning Is Recovering from Kidney Transplant Surgery," *Jet,* January 19, 2004, 47–48.

2. As noted in earlier chapters, "nephrotic syndrome" is a term that arose in the first half of the twentieth century to describe the association of heavy leakage of protein (mostly albumin) into the urine by the kidneys, edema (salt and water retention), decreased albumin in the blood (owing to the renal loss), and also elevated lipids in the blood, a secondary phenomenon that remains poorly understood. Nephrotic syndrome occurs with certain diseases of the kidneys that dominantly involve the glomeruli.

3. For a synopsis of information about FSGS and the filtering structure of the glomerulus as of 2006, see Julie Lin, "Focal Segmental Glomerulosclerosis," *Nephrology Rounds* 4, 5 (May 2006): n.p., available on www.nephrologyrounds.org; and Duncan Johnstone and Lawrence Holzman, "Clinical Impact of Research on the Podocyte Slit Diaphragm," *Nature Clinical Practice Nephrology* 2 (2006): 271–82.

4. As of 2006, most cases of FSGS are idiopathic—of unknown origin. A similar form of glomerular disease can occur, however, as an occasional complication of heroin addiction, extreme obesity, and certain disorders of the urinary tract in infancy.

5. Steven J. Peitzman, "Nephrology in America from Thomas Addis to the Artificial Kidney," in Russell C. Maulitz and Diana E. Long, eds., *Grand Rounds: One Hundred Years of Internal Medicine in America* (Philadelphia: University of Pennsylvania Press, 1988), 211–41 (an earlier version appeared as "Nephrology in the United States from Osler to the Artificial Kidney," *Annals of Internal Medicine* 105 [1986]: 937–46).

6. I refer to men because the research nephrologists of the period were in fact male, as few women had access to senior faculty positions in academic medicine. However, within each of the major laboratories were women scientists and technologists who made essential contributions. See Mabel Purkerson and Lilla Verkerdy, "History of Women in Nephrology (1918 to 1980)," *Seminars in Nephrology* 19 (1999): 89–94.

7. This ideology was formulated particularly by James Shannon, an early and perhaps the most influential NIH director. Before joining the NIH Shannon had in fact worked on basic renal physiology with Homer W. Smith of New York, one of the most important of renal physiologists. The phrase "of scientists by scientists" is from Cassious Van Slyke, "New Horizons in Medical Research," *Science* 104 (1946): 559–76, quote on p. 559. Van Slyke was the first director of the NIH extramural grants program.

8. Barry M. Brenner, Timothy Meyer, and Thomas Hostetter, "Dietary Protein Intake and the Progressive Nature of Kidney Disease: The Role of Hemodynamically Mediated Glomerular Injury in the Pathogenesis of Progressive Glomerular Sclerosis in Aging, Renal Ablation, and Intrinsic Renal Disease," *New England Journal of Medicine* 307 (1982): 652–59.

9. Brenner's group had identified a strain of rats, some of whose glomeruli were found on the surface of the kidney, making micropuncture of them feasible. For a brief interview with Brenner in which he recalls this work, see *Your Medicine Online,* an online newsletter of the Peter Bent Brigham Hospital from December 2004, at www.brighamandwomens.org/dom_newsletter/December_04/Brenner_Interview. htm (accessed July 31, 2006).

10. I have greatly simplified the emergence of this model. Tetsuo Shimamura and Ashton B. Morrison showed the probable relationship of compensatory hyperfiltration to sclerosis and obliteration of glomeruli ("A Progressive Glomerulosclerosis Occurring in Partial Five-sixths Nephrectomized Rats," *American Journal of Pathology* 79 [1975]: 95–106). See also Thomas H. Hostetter, Helmut G. Rennke, and Barry M. Brenner, "The Case for Intrarenal Hypertension in the Initiation and Progression of Diabetic and other Glomerulopathies," *American Journal of Medicine* 72 (1982): 375–80. An anthology of review papers dealing with reviving ideas on "progression" of chronic renal disease is William E. Mitch, ed., *The Progressive Nature of Renal Disease* (New York: Churchill Livingstone, 1986).

11. Subsequently, it has been established that effective blood pressure control in general retards the worsening of chronic renal disease, especially the proteinuric forms.

12. Saulo Klahr et al. (for the Modification of Diet in Renal Disease Study Group), "The Effects of Dietary Protein Restriction and Blood-Pressure Control on the Progression of Chronic Renal Disease," *New England Journal of Medicine* 330 (1994): 877–84.

13. Lionel Opie and Helmut Kowolik, "The Discovery of Captopril: From Large Animals to Small Molecules," *Cardiovascular Research* 30 (1995): 18–25.

14. The literature is huge. For some overviews, see, e.g., Tazeen Jafar et al., "Angiotensin-Converting Enzyme Inhibitors and Progression of Nondiabetic Renal

Disease," *Annals of Internal Medicine* 135 (2001): 73–87; Giuseppe Remuzzi et al., "Chronic Renal Diseases: Renoprotective Benefits of Renin-Angiotensin System Inhibition," *Annals of Internal Medicine* 136 (2002): 604–15; Lee Herbert, "Optimizing ACE-Inhibitor Therapy for Chronic Kidney Disease," *New England Journal of Medicine* 354 (2006): 189–91; Nitin Khosla and George Bakris, "Lessons Learned from Recent Hypertension Trials about Kidney Disease," *Clinical Journal of the American Society of Nephrology* 1 (2006): 229–35. All or most outpatient dialysis units in fact have the services of a nutritionist. Once a person is on dialysis, the dietary goals are adequate (not low) protein, some restriction on salt and potassium, and some limit on foods rich in phosphates.

15. A minority viewpoint held that it was merely effective lowering of blood pressure by the ACE inhibitors, and certain unfavorable renal effects of another class of antihypertensive drugs against which they were compared, that led to the seeming "renoprotective" benefit; see Anil Bidani and Karen Griffin, "The Benefits of Renin-Angiotensin Blockade in Hypertension Are Dependent on Blood-Pressure Lowering," *Nature Clinical Practice Nephrology* 2 (2006): 542–43.

16. Josef Coresh et al., "Chronic Kidney Disease Awareness, Prevalence, and Trends among U.S. Adults, 1999 to 2000," *Journal of the American Society of Nephrology* 16 (2005): 180–88.

17. Roland Blantz, "Reflections on the Past, Transitions to the Future: The American Society of Nephrology," *Journal of the American Society of Nephrology* 14 (2003): 1695–1703, quote on p. 1701.

18. National Kidney Foundation, "K/DOQI Clinical Practice Guidelines for Chronic Kidney Disease," published as supplement 1 of the *American Journal of Kidney Diseases* 39 (2002): S1–S266. These guidelines, including updates and additions, may also be found on the extensive Web site of the National Kidney Foundation, www.kidney.org.

19. Epoetin will not adequately stimulate blood production by the marrow unless the body contains adequate stores of iron, which is a key constituent of red cells.

20. Phosphate binders are medications that people on dialysis and some persons with renal disease prior to dialysis require to prevent the excess absorption of phosphate from their diet. Neither impaired kidneys nor the artificial ones excrete phosphate well, and a buildup in the body can lead to bone disease and other complications.

21. The finding of albumin in the urine would also declare that a person has CKD, even if his or her filtration rate remained normal.

22. This council included as members the National Kidney Foundation, the American Society of Nephrology, the Renal Physicians Association, the American Society of Transplantation, the Polycystic Kidney Disease Foundation, and the American Society of Pediatric Nephrology. See Thomas Parker et al., "The Chronic Kidney Disease Initiative," *Journal of the American Society of Nephrology* 15 (2004): 708–16.

23. "Stage 1" of CKD refers to albuminuria without loss of filtering capacity (elevated creatinine).

24. William Couser, "ISN and the 'New Nephrology,'" *Nature Clinical Practice Nephrology* 2 (2006): 541.

25. Allan Collins et al., "World Kidney Day: An Idea Whose Time Has Come," *Journal of the American Society of Nephrology* 17 (2006): 600–601. See also the Internet site for the International Federation of Kidney Foundations at www.ifkf.net.

26. Of course, physicians of the twentieth and twenty-first centuries would argue that their diuretic pills actually work, and through knowable mechanisms. But it is entirely possible that some of the plant and mercurial agents used in earlier times did produce some diuretic effect.

27. Richard Bright, "Cases and Observations Illustrative of Renal Disease Accompanied with Secretion of Albuminous Urine," *Guy's Hospital Reports* 1 (1836): 338–79, quotes on p. 338. The article is reprinted in *Original Papers of Richard Bright on Renal Disease*, ed. A. Arnold Osman (London: Oxford University Press, 1937), 93–131.

28. Evaluating and treating perturbations in the balance of acids and bases, salt and water, and potassium have been an important part of nephrology consultation practice in the hospital, even for disorders not caused by a renal disease. Much of the knowledge of these disorders, as well as the relevant normal physiology, has been developed by physicians and physiologists with special interest in the kidney.

INDEX

Readers using the index should be aware of the considerable overlap among the following names applied to generalized disorders of the kidney: Bright's Disease, chronic kidney disease, end-stage renal disease, glomerulonephritis, nephrotic syndrome, and proteinuria.

Page numbers in *italics* refer to illustrations.